DR PATRICIA GILBERT trained at St George's
Hospital Medical School, London, and has worked in
hospital and general practice in London and latterly
for the Community Health Service in south Warwick-
shire. She was also the clinical tutor and visiting
senior lecturer at Warwick University for a number of
years. Writing is now a full-time occupation for Dr
Gilbert; her most recent publications are *Helping
Children with Attention Deficit Disorder*, *Living with
Osteoarthritis* (both published by Sheldon Press) and
a textbook for nursery nurses. She is married with two
daughters.

Overcoming Common Problems Series

Selected titles
A full list of titles is available from Sheldon Press,
36 Causton Street, London SW1P 4ST, and on our website at
www.sheldonpress.co.uk

Assertiveness: Step by Step
Dr Windy Dryden and Daniel Constantinou

The Assertiveness Handbook
Mary Hartley

Breaking Free
Carolyn Ainscough and Kay Toon

Calm Down
Paul Hauck

The Candida Diet Book
Karen Brody

Cataract: What You Need to Know
Mark Watts

The Chronic Fatigue Healing Diet
Christine Craggs-Hinton

Cider Vinegar
Margaret Hills

Comfort for Depression
Janet Horwood

Confidence Works
Gladeana McMahon

Coping Successfully with Pain
Neville Shone

Coping Successfully with Panic Attacks
Shirley Trickett

Coping Successfully with Period Problems
Mary-Claire Mason

Coping Successfully with Prostate Cancer
Dr Tom Smith

Coping Successfully with Ulcerative Colitis
Peter Cartwright

Coping Successfully with Your Hiatus Hernia
Dr Tom Smith

Coping Successfully with Your Irritable Bowel
Rosemary Nicol

Coping with Alopecia
Dr Nigel Hunt and Dr Sue McHale

Coping with Anxiety and Depression
Shirley Trickett

Coping with Blushing
Dr Robert Edelmann

Coping with Bowel Cancer
Dr Tom Smith

Coping with Brain Injury
Maggie Rich

Coping with Candida
Shirley Trickett

Coping with Chemotherapy
Dr Terry Priestman

Coping with Childhood Allergies
Jill Eckersley

Coping with Childhood Asthma
Jill Eckersley

Coping with Chronic Fatigue
Trudie Chalder

Coping with Coeliac Disease
Karen Brody

Coping with Cystitis
Caroline Clayton

Coping with Depression and Elation
Patrick McKeon

Coping with Down's Syndrome
Fiona Marshall

Coping with Dyspraxia
Jill Eckersley

Coping with Eating Disorders and Body Image
Christine Craggs-Hinton

Coping with Eczema
Dr Robert Youngson

Coping with Endometriosis
Jo Mears

Coping with Epilepsy
Fiona Marshall and
Dr Pamela Crawford

Coping with Fibroids
Mary-Claire Mason

Coping with Gout
Christine Craggs-Hinton

Coping with Heartburn and Reflux
Dr Tom Smith

Coping with Incontinence
Dr Joan Gomez

Overcoming Common Problems Series

Overcoming Common Problems Series

Overcoming Common Problems Series

Overcoming Common Problems Series

Overcoming Common Problems

Coping with Macular Degeneration

Dr Patricia Gilbert

sheldon**PRESS**

First published in Great Britain in 2006

Sheldon Press
36 Causton Street
London SW1P 4ST

The author and publisher have made every effort to ensure that the external
website and email addresses included in this book are correct and up to date at
the time of going to press. The author and publisher are not responsible for the
content, quality or continuing accessibility of the sites.

British Library Cataloguing-in-Publication Data

A catalogue record for this book is available from the British Library

ISBN-13: 978–0–85969–943–3
ISBN-10: 0–85969–943–9

1 3 5 7 9 10 8 6 4 2

Typeset by Deltatype Limited, Birkenhead, Merseyside
Printed in Great Britain by
Ashford Colour Press

Contents

Acknowledgements

My thanks are due to Dr Sue Church for reading the manuscript and for her useful suggestions. Without her helpful encouragement and also that of the members of the local Macular Degeneration Society together with a number of friends who suffer from age-related macular degeneration (AMD) this text would have been the poorer. Their cheerful acceptance of the limitations imposed by AMD, together with practical hints on ways of coping have been humbling.

It is hoped that some of the ideas will be of value to others with this condition and that continuing research will soon find ways of prevention and successful treatment of this disease that is becoming more prevalent.

Introduction

Loss of vision can be one of our worst fears. Sadly, as we age, this does become more likely. In the early middle years reading difficulties frequently become apparent. (How often do youngsters wonder why ageing relatives are seen to be holding reading material at arm's length?) The cause of this is the lack of ability of the eyes at this time of life to adapt to the differing required lengths of vision. Corrective lenses will be the answer to this common problem.

Both long and short sight, if severe enough, will also need correction with lenses.

The cause of both these conditions is an anatomical one, and depends on the shape of the eye making the rays of light focus inappropriately on the retina. Both long and short sight can be present from an early age. It can often be seen to be genetically determined. For example, short sight can frequently be traced back through many generations. Fortunately today there are a wide variety of attractive frames to hold the lenses specific to each individual.

These facets of vision do not come into the category of visual loss – at least in those parts of the world where correction with appropriate lenses is commonplace and easily obtainable. True visual loss occurs when lenses of whatever type cannot return vision to normal.

There are many reasons for visual loss, and most of them are more common in later life. One of these is age-related macular degeneration – the subject of this book. (Macular degeneration can occur at any age, but is far less common than that occurring among older people – hence the name age-related macular degeneration or AMD. The following descriptions will relate to AMD. Where there are significant differences for younger people this will be explained.)

Vision can be arbitrarily divided into two parts – central

vision and peripheral vision. Central vision is that part of the visual field concerned with the seeing of objects immediately ahead. This applies to both distant objects and also to the visualization of those nearer tasks, such as reading, writing, sewing and the many other activities which require good close vision. Peripheral vision is that part of the visual field of which we are more dimly aware. Even when concentrating on the immediate view ahead, there is much that can be seen faintly and of which we become aware at the edges of a discrete view. Both aspects are important in normal visual acuity as will be seen later.

Central vision is the concern of a tiny specific area of the retina known as the macula, no bigger than a pin's head. It is when there is a degenerative process occurring that central vision is diminished or lost.

As with all problems of sight, it is important that an early and accurate diagnosis is made as to the cause. This must be done before any help or treatment can be given.

While AMD is at present not curable there are many ways in which aid can be given to make life easier. It is hoped that these pages will give information to both sufferers from AMD and to relatives and friends who do so much to help with those daily tasks that are proving difficult.

1

Working, and care, of the eye

The eye has been described as the 'window of the soul', and this part of the human body can indeed be a most expressive one. It has, however, a definite structure and physical function that can be mapped exactly. To be sure that this delicate organ remains in good working order for as long as possible, it is important that care is taken throughout life, and help obtained quickly if there should be any deterioration in vision.

Eyes are delicate spherical organs situated within a ring of bone known as the orbit. This firm ring consists of the cheekbone below, part of the skull above and the nasal bones between the two eyes. This beautifully made and specially adapted socket serves to protect the soft vulnerable tissue making up the eyeball. Accidents can of course involve the eyes, but without this bony protection much more frequent and dangerous damage could be done.

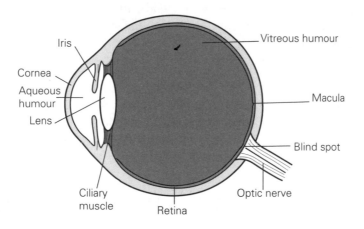

Figure 1 Cross-section of the human eye

From the diagram, the eye is seen to be shaped rather like a slightly elongated round ball, with a small bulge at the front. This latter part is known as the cornea. Beneath the cornea lies the iris, the coloured part of the eye which is unique to each individual and varies from very dark brown or black to the lightest of blue or green.

In the centre of the iris can be seen the pupil, a round black aperture. This pupil contracts and expands in response to the amount of light entering the eye at any one time. In bright light the pupil will become small to limit the amount of light entering. Conversely, when the light is dim the pupil will expand to allow more light to enter.

Behind the iris lies the lens. This has a jelly-like consistency contained within a capsule. This part of the eye changes shape allowing light rays to be focused accurately on the retina.

This retina is the all-important 'seeing' part of the eye, much like the film in a camera. It has specialized types of cells known as 'rods' and 'cones' with an underlying network of blood vessels and nerves which pass images of the outside world to the part of the brain concerned with the processing of vision and the subsequent interpretation of what is being visualized. The 'rods' are concerned with vision in dim light, while the 'cones' are concerned with the sharp sight needed in bright light.

The macula is that part of the retina which is concerned with

- seeing with clarity the objects straight ahead;
- the fine discrimination which allows us to perform so many small intricate tasks that are a part of everyday life;
- the visualization of colour.

This vital part of the retina, in spite of having such a vital function, is tiny. It measures only around 3 mm by 4 mm. A special pigment within the cells makes it appear a yellow colour.

The macula has a higher concentration of 'cones' than any

other part of the retina and also has a highly specialized blood and nerve supply. The cells are arranged in a specific pattern, rather like the hairs on a dog's coat or the pile on a piece of velvet – all pointing in one direction, towards the incoming light. Specific nerve fibres, up to one million, connect the macula to the ophthalmic part of the brain situated at the back of the head. Around 80 per cent of these nerve fibres are concerned with images coming from the macula. In this way the amount of information about the world is massive, and amounts to an extremely large part of how the world is viewed. In fact, more messages reach the brain from the macula than from any other separate part of the body.

So it can be seen what an enormous part in our understanding of the world the macula plays.

The optic nerve correlates all the incoming messages on their passage to the brain. This important structure is situated at the back of the eye, a little below the mid-line. Where this nerve enters the eye the smooth coating of the retina is necessarily interrupted. This gives rise to a 'blind spot', from which signals from the outside world are not received. Probably everyone at some time or other has been aware of the existence of this blind spot. Objects can be seen to come into the field of vision in a most unexpected way when they have for a short while previously been quite invisible. Care needs to be taken to be aware of the existence of a blind spot when driving and looking out for traffic coming from behind.

The whole eyeball behind the lens is filled with a viscous fluid know as the vitreous humour. The smaller chamber in front of the lens is similarly filled with fluid of a slightly more watery nature known as the aqueous humour. These jelly-like substances ensure that the eyeball keeps its smooth, rounded shape.

Attached to each side of the eyeball are the extra-ocular muscles concerned with the movement of the eye in all directions. It is when these muscles function abnormally, due to a number of reasons, that a squint is obvious. Two further tiny muscles, the ciliary muscles, situated near the iris, control

3

the altering shape of the lens as it adapts to visualize objects at differing distances.

Visits to the optometrist

These visits should be made on a regular basis – every two years is a good interval – to ensure eye health. Obviously earlier visits will be necessary if there are any visual problems or difficulties.

Children are not seen as regularly by opticians as are adults. Vision in the younger age group is monitored as part of the ongoing developmental checks throughout childhood. Any problems are then usually referred to an ophthalmologist (a doctor who specializes in visual problems who usually works in a hospital or special clinic), such as the rare macular degeneration seen in children. Squints or the rare macular problems are the most common reasons for further investigation.

Squints

Squints are especially important to be checked out in children. Lack of early treatment can result in impaired vision in one eye later in life. The cause of a squint may be the simple one of a refractive error (long or short sight) in just one eye. This can result in blurred, or even double, vision. If this is uncorrected the visual pathways to the brain can fail to develop adequately with the result that the vision is less than perfect in one eye. This situation is often referred to as a 'lazy' eye. Squints can also occur in adults for a variety of medical reasons. (Squints are a fascinating subject in themselves, but are outside the scope of this book.)

Ageing

Around the 40-year-old age mark many people find they need the services of an optometrist. It is at this age that small print becomes more and more difficult to read, as well as problems with other forms of close work. This is due to a decrease in the ability of the extra-ocular muscles to pull the eye into a position to focus properly on the print – to 'accommodate' to the differing situation. This is known as 'presbyopia'. Also, with advancing years, the lens tends to lose its elasticity and so, again, accommodation becomes less efficient.

Brief overview of routine checks

The following are a selection of the conditions routinely checked at a visit to an optician (or optometrist). Following on from checking as to why an appointment has been made, much can be learnt from asking about any medical or family history. For example, some drugs used for other medical conditions may affect vision. Any previous, or recent, injury to the eye (even a small amount of dust rubbed into an eye, perhaps forgotten) can cause damage.

From the point of view of macular degeneration found in children or young people it is important to ask about any family history of visual difficulties. Juvenile macular degeneration has a more direct genetic inheritance than the age-related type. Cousin marriages – more usual in closed communities – can be of importance when considering the possible genetic background.

Visual acuity

The first check done tests what actually can be seen, both near and long sight. For the testing of long sight the familiar Snellen Chart, with letters of differing sizes is used, each eye being tested separately. Close vision is then checked by reading from a standardized reading type book. From around middle age on, the majority of people require spectacles for reading. (This 'presbyopia' is a normal ageing process.)

Reaction of the pupil

The size, and the reaction, of the pupils to light can give clues to various other possible medical conditions elsewhere in the body. For example, a difference in size between the two pupils can point to a possible nerve problem and the relatively rare condition of a small pupil together with a drooping eyelid can raise suspicions of disease elsewhere in the body. Dilated pupils are sometimes found in very short-sighted people, and small pupils are often seen in babies or older people.

Corneal abrasions

If there has been any recent history of an injury, however slight, to the eye the possibility of a corneal abrasion, or graze, should be considered. This is where something in the eye can cause an injury to the delicate outer part of the cornea. It is of importance that even a minor degree of trauma should be treated to prevent scarring of the cornea which would permanently affect vision. With the insertion of special fluorescent drops into the eye any abrasion will be clearly seen.

Glaucoma

This is a condition in which the pressure inside the eyeball becomes too high due to lack of drainage of fluid. This condition can come on acutely and rapidly with green haloes being seen round light and pain in the eye. It is more usual, however, for the condition to arise slowly, and the sufferer only to be aware of what is happening when vision begins to deteriorate. A special instrument is used to check this pressure. Only a small puff of air is felt as the instrument is applied to the eye.

Field of vision

If there is any doubt as to specific parts of the normal visual field being missed, a field of vision test is done. With macular degeneration it is the middle part of the visual field that is affected. Other conditions can affect different part of this field, for instance, glaucoma will affect a different part of the visual field from that affected by macular degeneration.

Ophthalmoscopy

This is the process whereby the optometrist examines the back of the eye with an instrument known as an ophthalmoscope. The room is darkened and a view of the structures at the back of the eye is obtained when you are asked to focus on a small red light. (This is merely to keep the eye as still as possible – quite difficult to do, as it is an automatic reaction to look away from a bright light.) Occasionally, if there is thought to be a problem at the back of the eye, drops to dilate the pupil are instilled. These take around 20 minutes to act, but a much better and more comprehensive view of the back of the eye can then be obtained. (Following the instillation of the dilating drops, vision is misty for around an hour, and it is wise to have some help in getting home after this has been done. Driving should certainly not be attempted. Sunlight, too, will appear extra bright, so it is a good idea to take along a pair of sunglasses to wear for an hour or two.)

The above is a brief run-down of the usual elements in a routine eye examination. Obviously if there are any more complicated problems, further specialized tests will be necessary – see later in the book. Digital cameras now play an important and splendid part in visualizing the back of the eye in minute detail. With this equipment, the state of the blood vessels in the eye as well as other potential problems can be seen.

Summary

- Anatomy and physiology of the eye.
- Visits to the optometrist.
- Routine checks.

2
What is age-related macular degeneration?

As mentioned earlier the retina is that part of the eye most intimately concerned with the processing of visual images. All other structures of the eye – the pupil, lens, vitreous fluid, for example – focus onto and supply this camera-like surface.

The basic structure of the retina consists of an intricate network of fine nerves, blood vessels and the rods and cones vital for vision. Blood vessels in any part of the body provide nourishment by way of a wide variety of gases and many vital trace elements. They also carry away, for further recycling and processing, the waste products of metabolism. This is as true of the blood vessels which supply the retina as in any other organ of the body.

We have seen that the macula is the all-important part of the retina when it comes to good central vision. Situated in the centre of the back of the globe of the eye in line with the pupil and the lens, it is ideally placed to view and process objects and scenes immediately ahead. It is here that the fine details of nature such as the delicate lines on a leaf vein, the perfect shape of a flower bud or the ever-changing waves of the sea are enjoyed. Here, too, the changing expressions on someone's face can be noted. Again this is the place where all the differing shades of colour are appreciated. All these nuances of daily living which enhance existence as well as giving help with the understanding of thoughts and feelings are due to the clear images to be found on the macula.

In age-related macular degeneration (AMD) this important layer of the retina begins to deteriorate. As this progresses the previously sharp images of central vision become less and less effective. Vision straight ahead becomes progressively blurred until, over time, the whole of the central vision is blotted out.

It is only this central area of vision that is affected in AMD. Peripheral vision – i.e. all the surrounding areas of vision of which we are usually more dimly aware are unaffected. So, most importantly, total vision is not lost in AMD – very much diminished and certainly handicapping, but nevertheless a certain amount of visual independence can be maintained throughout life. Much help, with low-vision aids, adaptations to daily living and understanding of the problems of lack of central vision can be given to make life with AMD as little of a burden as possible. (See later chapters on ways of coping.)

Types of AMD

'Dry' AMD

Depending on the type of macular degeneration occurring, visual loss varies in the rate of progression. With dry AMD the loss of vision occurs gradually over many months or years. Indeed it can be thought that the increasingly poor vision is due to a general increase in presbyopia (the reading difficulty so frequently experienced in middle age and afterwards). So it is important that a visit to an optometrist is made if there are concerns on this score. Being aware of potential problems can make an early diagnosis possible so that treatment and coping strategies can be organized.

Dry AMD is the most common form of the condition and occurs in around 90 per cent of sufferers. This type occurs when there is a lack of adequate nutrition and a build-up of waste materials in the macular region of the retina. This is due to the inability of the blood vessels to carry out their vital function of supplying and removing metabolic substances.

On looking at the macular region of the retina with an ophthalmoscope it can be seen why vision has been so affected by the disease. If AMD is present this area is seen to be covered with a fatty, yellowish substance, rather like scrambled egg. This is the final result of the failure of the underlying blood vessels to carry out their function of removing the waste materials of metabolism. So it can be readily understood why vision is blurred and interrupted when light rays fail to penetrate this mass of unwanted material, known as 'drusen'.

Dry AMD does not always mean that reading skills are totally lost. With adequate magnification and good lighting reading can still be possible – not without some degree of difficulty but nevertheless this skill which forms so much a part of daily living is not entirely lost.

'Wet' AMD

This occurs when a mass of tiny new blood vessels grow behind the macular area of the retina. These blood vessels are weak and function abnormally. Instead of containing blood and fluid within their walls, leakage of fluid occurs into the surrounding tissue. In this way the macular region is damaged and scarred. This results in loss of vision.

With this type of AMD the visual loss occurs more rapidly than with the dry type. Around 10 per cent of people suffer from this wet type. It is important that this type of AMD is diagnosed early. Treatment can be tried if the condition is found to be at an early stage. Possibly because of a delay in diagnosis and hence the time lost in giving treatment wet AMD can give rise to the worst scenario for visual loss. But some cases are suitable for specific treatment which can halt the progression of the disease.

This will depend on which subsection of the type of wet AMD is present. The 'classic' type occurs when the abnormal blood vessels are within the retina. The 'occult' type occurs when the abnormal vessels are hidden deep under the retina.

Macular degeneration frequently affects both eyes, but it is usual for vision in one eye to be diminished before the other eye is affected. Understandably this can lead to a delay in diagnosis. The unaffected eye compensates for the visual loss in the affected eye and so reduced vision can pass unnoticed for some time – often many months or even years. If only one eye has been diagnosed as having AMD there can be concern about using the unaffected eye excessively, but this will not affect the onset of problems in this much used eye. Eyes are

11

not 'worn out' by constant use, so full advantage needs to be taken of the good vision in the unaffected eye.

For the above reason it is so important that each eye is looked at and tested separately when visiting an optometrist. Again an important reason for regular eye checks – every two years or sooner if any visual difficulties are noticed. (At present in the UK checks of vision are free for citizens over the age of 60 years, and for certain other people, such as those who have a first-degree relative with glaucoma. Prescription lenses and frames do, however, have to be paid for.)

Summary

- It is only central vision that is lost in age-related macular degeneration.
- Peripheral vision is unaffected.
- There are two types of AMD – 'dry' and 'wet'.
- Treatment is potentially possible for the 'wet' type.
- Both eyes can be affected, within different time spans.
- Regular eye tests are important later in life.

3

The numbers game and risk factors

Age-related macular degeneration (AMD) is probably not as well known or documented as a cause of visual loss as is, for example, cataract or glaucoma. These latter conditions are the subject of much conversation among older people as they are the group most affected by both these conditions.

A reason for the probable greater knowledge of cataract and glaucoma, for example, is that there are well-known treatments available. At present there are no known methods of cure for AMD – apart from the success of laser treatment for the select few people with the wet form of AMD. But it must be remembered that much can be done to make life more bearable for people with AMD.

AMD is a condition which is not painful – unlike glaucoma at times. So the onset of AMD may well not be considered to be an urgent reason to contact a doctor or optician. There is nothing like pain to send anyone off for help!

AMD is the leading cause for registered blindness – or partially sighted in many cases – in the UK and USA. There are over 200,000 known cases of registered visual loss due to AMD in the UK. It is thought that this is only the tip of the iceberg. There are probably many more people with the condition who have not as yet been diagnosed – for a variety of reasons, the lack of regular visual checks being one of the most common. This is understandable with the dry type of AMD as the deterioration in visual acuity can be slow. One can almost hear the more mature person of over 60 saying, 'I just need new glasses – I'll have my eyes checked when I have time.' Well, maybe they do just need some adjustment to their reading spectacles, but maybe not. It is always wise to check on this at an early stage rather than later.

Again, AMD being such a relatively unknown condition, the index of suspicion is low when visual acuity begins to deteriorate. It is to be hoped that with more knowledge of this condition being available a greater, and quicker, diagnosis will occur so that immediate help can be set in motion.

It must also be remembered that in the West longevity is becoming more common. So, with this increase in years, the incidence of AMD will undoubtedly also increase. Of necessity this will also increase the rate of research into treatments and coping strategies as more and more people are affected. Yet again an important reason for having regular eye checks as one matures. But even taking into account this increase in an older population, there is some evidence that the actual incidence of age-related macular degeneration is on the increase.

Worldwide the picture is even more daunting. It is thought that up to 30 million people are affected to some degree by some form of AMD. This is a sizeable number and one which, considering that many of these sufferers have little or no access to help with their disability, could have effects on economic growth.

More unusually, macular degeneration can affect people of a younger, working age. This will, of course, pose added problems of coping with the disease on the working life ahead.

Risk factors

While the actual cause of AMD is unknown at present, there are some factors which would seem to point to a greater risk of the disease occurring in some people.

These risk factors are not strictly definitive. Just because one or more risk factors for a certain disease or condition apply to an individual does not mean that they will inevitably suffer from this condition. Of course, when several of the risk factors are present the chances will be greater. While the cause of AMD is unknown, it is probably necessary that a number of factors working together determines whether or not the condition becomes fully manifest. Fortunately, although some risk factors – as for any illness or condition – are quite beyond our control, there are other points over which we can have control to exert a beneficial effect. AMD, as with many other diseases, does have this split. So let us look first at the unmodifiable conditions that may predispose us to AMD.

Factors which cannot be modified

Age

By definition age-related macular degeneration is a condition which occurs in the over-50s or more commonly in the over-60s. Regretfully there is nothing at all that can be done – at present anyway – to alter the ageing process. (As mentioned previously macular degeneration is not entirely unknown in younger age groups, but this has a genetic basis. Macular degeneration is very much a condition of older people.)

Genetics

We all inherit characteristics from both our parents. Some are directly passed on by the laws of inheritance, such as eye colour, height and general body configuration (and many others, including a number of specific diseases). These characteristics can readily be seen in a photograph of many family members.

There are also family traits that are not directly passed on, but which rather lead to a tendency towards certain traits. Examples of this can be a hot temper or a placid nature, an optimistic attitude to life or one which is filled with gloom and doom – and there are a multitude of others which can readily be thought of.

The tendency to certain diseases can also be seen to work in a similar way, and the tendency to AMD is no exception. If there are one or more family members suffering from the condition, the chances are greater for younger members, as they age, to also be affected. Genetics play a larger part in macular degeneration in younger people.

In this context first-degree marriages – i.e. first cousins –

15

make it more likely that early macular degeneration could occur if the susceptibility is already present in the genes.

Again there is nothing that can be done to modify this one factor.

Gender

We have no way of choosing our gender, although parents in the future may have this opportunity. Women are more at risk of suffering from AMD than men. At 75 years of age, or over, there are around twice as many women as men with AMD. Why this is so is not clear, although hormone balance may have something to do with this.

Long sight

People who can see clearly into the distance are said to be long-sighted. These are those people who will usually need reading glasses at an earlier age than their short-sighted brothers or sisters – that is those whose near vision is excellent but who have more difficulty visualizing objects in the far distance.

Long sight, which depends to a large extent on the actual size and shape of the eye is often a directly inherited characteristic. This is not such a definitive characteristic for the onset of AMD, but one which does at times seem to have a bearing. Some reports also suggest that short sight, too, may be a disposing factor. Not perhaps as marked as the risks of developing glaucoma, but nevertheless a factor to be considered (see section on glaucoma in Chapter 6).

Race

Macular degeneration is found primarily in fair-skinned, blue-eyed people. Races with dark skins do not suffer from this form of visual problem.

The above factors are those over which we have no control. We are unable to choose our parents with all their good or bad characteristics. Similarly we are unable to choose our sex, our predisposition, or otherwise, to refractive errors.

But fortunately there are some factors, which are also thought to have a bearing on the possibility of suffering from AMD, over which we can exert some influence.

Factors which can be modified

Diet

Diet is, and has been for some time, the subject of discussion in the onset of many diseases. Diets, good and bad, fill much space in today's newspapers and magazines.

The incidence of many diseases has been laid at the door of an inadequate, or insufficient diet, rightly or wrongly. Diet is also considered to possibly have some bearing on the incidence of AMD in a specific way. In many foodstuffs and the products of their breakdown are oxygen charged molecules known as 'free radicals'. These free radicals, if present in the body in excess, are thought to cause damage to the macula leading to the deterioration seen in AMD.

The action of these rogue free radicals (and it is not only in the incidence of AMD, but also in some forms of cancer) can be counteracted by nutrients in the diet which have an antioxidant action. If the diet is low in these antioxidants, this may be a risk factor about which something can be done.

Research into diet and AMD has suggested that a diet high in carotenoids, which are powerful antioxidants, may help to prevent the onset of this condition. There are only two of the wide range of carotenoids to be found in the tissue of the macula – lutein and zeaxanthin. So it would seem that a diet which contains an adequate amount of these substances could be a modifiable factor in the chances of suffering from AMD.

Foodstuffs containing high levels of lutein and zeaxanthin are mainly those in green vegetables. Broccoli, kale, spinach and lettuce contain the highest levels, but peas, sprouts and green beans also have useful amounts. A serving of one or more of these vegetables two or three times a week could help reduce the risk of the onset of AMD. It is also thought that high dietary levels of these foodstuffs could slow the progress of existing AMD. So a slight alteration in diet, with the help of many of the delicious recipes that abound for so many foodstuffs these days, would be a small price to pay for the possibility of reducing the risk of AMD.

Smoking

Smoking not only increases the risk of both heart and lung diseases, but is also thought to be a factor in the onset of age-related macular degeneration. A recent piece of research concluded that AMD is twice as common in people who smoked more than 20 cigarettes a day as compared with non-smokers.

The way in which this happens is that smoking reduces the activity of the protective antioxidants. We have already seen that these are important factors in laying to rest the action of the destructive free radicals in the body. Better never to have smoked at all, but to stop as one matures is better than continuing to smoke – from many health points of view.

Much help is available to assist in giving up this habit. Also recent legislation limiting the places where smoking is permitted can help to overcome the habit.

Alcohol

To a lesser extent than smoking, but nevertheless one to be considered, is the excessive intake of alcohol on a daily basis. Again a reduction in the level of antioxidants is the key. There is no need to give up alcohol altogether, but it is advisable to stick to the recommended daily units. (An extra helping of green vegetables in lieu of a drink is not perhaps a wished for option, but perhaps a sensible one!)

Sunlight

Situated in the direct line of vision behind the lens of the eye, the macular region of the retina is especially susceptible to the action of sunlight. Damage to these highly sensitive cells can occur if excess sunlight over a prolonged period of time is focused on the eye.

People with light-coloured eyes – shades of blue and grey – are more liable to have a greater degree of sunlight focused on the macula. The darker colour of brown or black eyes will filter out much of the bright light of sunlight. Perhaps it can be postulated that light has something to do with the onset of macular degeneration.

Avoidance of sitting in bright sunlight for any length of time should be considered, but it is not necessary to stay out of bright sunlight altogether. Doing this will lose the beneficial effects of fine, sunny weather either in the long summer days or the bright frosty ones of winter. Rather it is a good idea to wear sunglasses – prescription ones if necessary – when in bright sunlight. Care needs to be taken when buying sunglasses. Those with the CE mark mean that they meet European quality standards. A wide-brimmed hat can also reduce the amount of bright light focused on the eye.

High blood pressure

It has been suggested that having untreated high blood pressure may be an added factor in the onset of AMD. While not proven, it is wise to have a blood pressure check on a regular basis, so that treatment can be given if necessary. High blood pressure has an effect on all the blood vessels in the body, and so it would seem that these blood vessels in the macula will not be excluded. General vascular problems do not in themselves cause macular degeneration, but it is probable that generalized abnormalities in this part of the body mechanism could have an added effect.

There are a number of relatively easy modifications that can be made to reduce, as far as is possible, the risk of AMD. So to summarize:

- Eat a diet high in antioxidants – green leafy vegetables.
- Stop smoking.
- Keep alcohol intake to reasonable limits.

- Take steps to limit the amount of direct sunlight entering the eye – wear sunglasses and wide-brimmed hats.
- Check on general health, including any vascular problems.

Summary

- Age-related macular degeneration is a leading cause of blindness, or partial sight, in people over 60 in the UK and USA.
- 20 to 30 million people worldwide are thought to be affected by some degree of macular degeneration.
- There are certain modifications that can help to reduce the risk.
- It is important to have regular eye checks.

4
Signs and symptoms of macular degeneration

So much for the incidence and risk factors for age-related macular degeneration (AMD). All rather theoretical perhaps, but how will this condition manifest itself in any one individual? This chapter gives information on tests that need to be done to ensure that any visual disturbances noticed are due to macular degeneration, and a later chapter gives brief descriptions of other common conditions in which visual loss or disturbance is present.

Early warning signs

Macular degeneration is a condition which does not occur suddenly. Other eye diseases, such as a retinal haemorrhage (as can occur in diabetic retinopathy), or a retinal detachment will give rise to a sudden partial or complete loss of sight. In contrast, macular degeneration makes itself known relatively slowly over months, and the signs may not be immediately noticeable or can be confused with other pre-existing eye problems. They can be put down to some aberration of the light, tiredness, a bout of general ill-health or genuinely not perceived as important.

There are five specific effects which may indicate that macular degeneration is a possible cause. Any one, or combination, of these signs should receive immediate attention from an eye clinic. The importance of early correct diagnosis cannot be overstressed. Although the dry type of AMD is incurable at present, it is possible to ameliorate some types of the wet type, and certainly to start important coping strategies. The sooner the diagnosis is made, the earlier these vital coping strategies can be instituted.

Shape

Differences in the shape of objects can be one of the first signs of AMD. The classic most often quoted alteration in shape is the apparent crookedness of an upright object, such as a lamp-post or window frame. These rigid straight objects will be seen as having a wavy or crooked bend along part of their structure. Horizontal everyday pieces of furniture or other household equipment will also be visualized as being crooked or having a wavy trend. (This was much in evidence in Gwendoline's story later in this chapter.)

If only one eye is affected, as can be the case in many early stages of macular degeneration, this effect can be disregarded by closing the affected eye, and viewing objects with one eye only. This trick, which can become almost automatic, will restore the crooked object to its usual shape.

It can readily be understood how misunderstanding about this facet of macular degeneration can happen. It is only when these effects become more frequent or occur in conjunction with other visual problems that it will be realized something serious is amiss.

This perceived alteration in shape is due to the altered, diseased, arrangement of the specialized cells in the macula. Light falling on 'crooked' cells will lead to 'crooked' vision.

Size

Perhaps less frequently than alterations in shape, alterations in size can be noticed. Objects ranging from a small teacup to a larger garden structure can be seen to be either larger or smaller. This can result in accidents in finding the exact position of everyday objects. For example, if a cup of tea is visualized as smaller than it really is reaching out for the handle can have disastrous consequences and lead to uninformed cries of clumsiness. This may be thought of as all part of ageing, when in reality it is a definitive visual problem.

Similarly stretching out to something that appears larger

than normal will result in fumbling when contact is not made when it is expected. Again this can all too easily be put down to the general disability of old age. It is possible that some of the falls so often sustained by older people could be due to some disturbance of vision.

Colour

The bright colours of nature and of everyday objects all around can also be affected by macular degeneration. Colours previously easily differentiated can prove impossible to distinguish between. An example of this is the difference between a black fabric and a dark navy blue one. (But in the artificial light of department stores this can prove almost impossible, even to those with good vision. Labels stating colour should be mandatory!) The choosing of brightly coloured clothing and furnishings may be due to the diminution in colour vision.

Younger sufferers from macular degeneration are more likely to be aware of the lack of colour discrimination than people with age-related macular degeneration. Could it be that this is because discriminating between colours is more a matter of memory than we realize in the older age group?

It is worth remembering that colour vision is not perfect in many people, especially in the male sex. As many as one in eight men have some degree of colour vision defect – the red/ green type being the most common. This problem should be picked up routinely during the school years. Defective colour vision can preclude boys from a number of possible careers, such as train drivers and pilots, for example. It is as well to be aware of this before the time comes to choose a career, to avoid devastating disappointment.

Flashing lights

This can be an unpleasant occasional experience in the early stages of macular degeneration. Whirling coloured flashes of bright light happen sporadically and seem especially common

23

in the twilight hours when just dropping off to sleep or wakening. Fortunately this is not a continuing process. This phenomenon will disappear as the disease progresses and the diseased cells causing the problem become unable to function.

Likewise driving at night can be difficult with the onset of macular degeneration. Oncoming headlights become like mini starbursts which linger. Again this can be put down to the ageing process, especially if spectacles are worn for driving. Night driving can be difficult for many people anyway, and the early symptoms of macular degeneration can compound the difficulties.

A darkened room or the wearing of sunglasses during daylight hours will do nothing to relieve the problem of these flashing lights, as it is the reaction of the diseased cells in the macula rather than a response to light entering the eye from the outside world.

Sunlight

In addition to the flashing lights described above, direct sunlight can also cause discomfort. Here sunglasses, or a green-coloured eye shield, can be helpful. The latter may be of more help than sunglasses. Sunglasses will reduce the light falling on the retina concerned with peripheral vision. This in turn will reduce the amount of available side vision. If sunglasses are chosen, it is important that they do what they are supposed to do – namely to cut out ultraviolet rays from the sun. These are the rays that can damage the retina and are thought to have some bearing possibly on the cause of macular degeneration, particularly in people with blue or light-coloured eyes. Remember, too, that ultraviolet rays are present even when the sun is not fully out. Clouds do not completely restrict these rays, especially at midday in the summer. So be sure to buy sunglasses from a reputable source. Prescription sunglasses, if correcting lenses are necessary, can be obtained from an optometrist.

And do not forget the benefits of a wide-brimmed hat for cutting down on sun glare.

If any of these signs is noticed – or any combination of them – it is vitally important that immediate advice is obtained. The optometrist or your GP can refer you to the local eye clinic, and do insist this is done as soon as possible. Treatment for some forms of macular degeneration needs to be given early. This condition should be regarded as an emergency.

The case history below highlights the problems that can be associated with the onset of macular degeneration in a woman who already had some visual difficulties. Confusion can easily arise, and needs specialized help to sort out.

Gwendoline

Gwendoline (and she disliked being called Gwen!) was 76 and had been a widow for 15 years. Until five years ago she had coped very adequately with life on her own. Having no children she had relied on friends to help with some of the everyday problems that inevitably arose during the course of the years. Visiting friends, playing bridge and driving to a wide variety of scenic locations in her small car had made life bearable following the death of her husband,

Her vision had not been good for many years as she was short-sighted. But spectacles had been prescribed which helped this common problem.

One eye in particular, however, had given her some problems a few years previously with an attack of temporal arteritis. This disease of the blood vessels had been held in check by medication with steroids. This drug had been gradually reduced over the years, but Gwendoline still needed a small dose daily.

It was when she was visiting a young neighbour that she realized that her vision was not as good as it had been a month or so previously. Susie's face was slightly blurred and Gwendoline found it difficult to decide just what colour sweater she was wearing. 'I must make an appointment with the optician soon,' she thought to herself. 'My glasses have not been checked for a while.'

But life at Christmastime became hectic with invitations

to stay with friends around the country. So Gwendoline put off checking on her eyesight. 'I can still see to drive,' she told herself. 'It's only this left eye that is being a bit of a problem.'

It was the day after Boxing Day that Gwendoline became really concerned – not just about her vision but with her ability to cope with life on her own. She was sitting quietly, thinking about the busy events of the past week, when she noticed that the skirting board beside her chair was not only wavy, but also appeared to be gradually moving. The curtains, too, did not appear to be hanging straight. She got up and gave them a tweak, and settled down to watch television for a time.

But it was no good. The skirting board with its wavy outline kept catching her attention. Also when she looked up at the lampshade, a blob of bright red appeared over the pale silk surface. This then disappeared, only to return again momentarily.

'Perhaps I've had just too much of a merry Christmas,' she thought wryly to herself, but basically knowing that this had not been so. She turned off the offending light and went slowly upstairs to bed.

The holiday period seemed to extend for ever and Gwendoline became more and more worried with the weird visual effects that seemed to be getting worse rather then improving. At times she was almost beginning to doubt her sanity. Living alone was no help to rational thought.

Fortunately she was able to make an appointment early in January with her usual optometrist. 'Perhaps it is the return of my temporal arteritis,' she said hesitantly. 'But it is the other eye that seems to be the problem now, and I certainly never had anything like this before.'

Gwendoline's optometrist listened carefully to her descriptions of wavy lines and flashing bursts of colour. 'Let's dilate your pupils, so I can have a good look at the back of your eyes,' he said comfortingly.

Twenty minutes later and Gwendoline's vision was misty

26

following the instillation of the dilating eye drops. The bright light of the ophthalmoscope flashed into her eye.

'It would seem that you have the beginnings of a problem with the macula in this eye,' she was told. 'It is important that this is checked out thoroughly at the eye clinic at the hospital.'

The optician went on to explain to Gwendoline what was causing the unusual visual effects that had been worrying her, and the possibility of macular degeneration was mentioned. Later on that week the ophthalmologist confirmed the optician's diagnosis of early age-related macular degeneration in Gwendoline's left eye.

While being shocked at this news, Gwendoline in some ways was relieved that the problem had not been due to either her imagination or her fears of losing her sanity. Subsequently, Gwendoline's macular degeneration was found to be of the dry type, about which little could be done at present.

But with much help and advice, Gwedoline is managing very well to cope with her visual problems. Her only regret is that her car has had to be sold as she is now not safe to drive. 'I'm less mobile now,' she has been heard to say, 'but I have so many good friends who ferry me around.'

This case history highlights the need for professional help in sorting out the diagnosis of visual problems. Just because Gwendoline had already suffered from one eye disease (temporal arteritis) this did not mean that the new symptoms were due to the same cause. Different symptoms need careful investigation to determine the exact cause of the current difficulty in seeing clearly.

Summary

- Macular degeneration comes on slowly, over months or years.
- Visual disturbance, such as changes in size, shape and colour are early signs.

- Difficulties with flashing lights or dislike of bright sunlight can also occur.
- It is vital that a diagnosis is made as soon as possible.

5
Testing for age-related macular degeneration

Before any examination of, or any specific tests on, the eye, the ophthalmologist will want to know exactly how vision is being affected. Clues can be gleaned from descriptions of differences in size, shape or colour.

In some ways, however, a history of the onset, symptoms and progression of the disease are not as vital as with disease in other parts of the body. It is fortunate that the eye can be examined relatively easily in minute detail by way of the ophthalmoscope (the piece of equipment which is used to look at the back of the eye).

Other parts of the body are not so readily accessible. Various procedures are necessary to take a look at any potentially diseased part. An example of this is the endoscopic examination of the oesophagus and stomach. Here a small camera is passed via the nose or throat in order to view these hidden organs.

In contrast most of the structures of the eye can be seen, and particularly so after the pupil has been dilated. As mentioned previously this is done by the instillation of special drops which temporarily paralyse the pupil in the dilated position. If this is not done the pupil would automatically constrict in reaction to any bright light falling onto the eye.

To test this for yourself – look in the mirror, cover one eye with a hand for a couple of minutes. On removing the darkening hand the pupil will be seen to constrict quickly as the light once more falls on the eye.

As the eye is so readily examined, a detailed history of the problem is not quite as important as with other diseases in other parts of the body where direct visualization is difficult or impossible. Nevertheless, enquiries into any family history of visual problems and especially anyone who in later life has macular degeneration is important and may help in the unravelling of the cause of this condition.

Genetic factors are less likely to be involved in AMD than in younger people who have the condition. For example, the type of macular degeneration known as Stargardt's disease (or juvenile macular dystrophy) usually shows itself in the second or third decades of life. This condition is inherited when both parents carry the abnormal gene. If only one parent carried this gene, children would not be affected, although they may be a 'carrier'. It is more likely that an abnormal gene occurs in both mother and father if they are blood-related. So enquiries about any intermarriage is worth while.

While inherited problems are more usual in the younger type of macular degeneration, genetic problems could possibly occur in the later age-related type. Environmental factors on top of a possible genetic predisposition may play a part. Research into the possible genetic input into eye diseases is ongoing, and this could help in the understanding of the cause of macular degeneration. Once this is understood, possible methods of treatment and/or prevention are a step nearer.

As we have seen, the most helpful investigation in the diagnosis of macular degeneration is the examination of the eye – first by testing what can actually be seen by the sufferer, and second by looking into the eye.

In testing the visual acuity, three main tests need to be done.

- Long distance vision is tested by the well-known Snellen Chart of various size letters. Depending on the stage of the disease, varying results will be obtained, and are often not especially helpful. But most helpful of all, and of which note should be immediately taken, is the throwaway remark that the examiner's face cannot be clearly seen – even though the surrounding furnishings are clear.
- Near vision then needs to be tested by means of reading different sized typefaces. Again, depending on the stage of the macular degeneration, results are variable. With

advanced macular degeneration only the reading matter on the periphery of the test card can be seen and that only with difficulty.

These two tests will quantify the level of vision.

One particular type of macular dysfunction is worth mentioning here. If much of the text can be read easily but the odd word or even letter is missing this can be a sign that only a very small part of the macula is involved. Possibly only a minute bubble of leaked fluid is occurring over this vital area of vision.

This is termed a 'macular hole', and is indicative that further degeneration may occur at a later date. (Missing letters, and sometimes whole words, can also occur in some people suffering from a specific type of migraine. But under these circumstances there will be other signs of migraine, such as headache, giddiness and/or nausea and vomiting.)

• Testing with the Amsler Chart. This is a chart consisting of a number of small squares with a well-defined dot in the centre. The lines of the square are quite straight, and are seen to be so by people with normal vision. On testing (each eye separately), focus must be made on the central dot. If macular degeneration is present the lines connecting the sides of the squares will appear to be bent, wavy or missing altogether. Also with normal vision it is possible to visualize all four corners of the square while concentrating on the middle dot. This test is not in common use, but can give warning signs that a visual problem is present or developing. But it is a good test for detecting early signs of macular degeneration.

Following these everyday tests, further examination with the ophthalmoscope will need to be done. As previously mentioned dilation of the pupil is necessary so that the bright light of the equipment does not cause the pupil to constrict and so prevent viewing of the structures at the back of the eye.

31

Drops will be gently instilled into both eyes. Over a space of around 20 minutes, vision will gradually become more and more blurred. Normally the pupil constricts and dilates according to the amount of light entering the eye and to fix the length of focus required for a variety of visual purposes. With the pupil fixed in the dilated position, this accommodation process becomes impossible. Everything can still be seen but will appear misty. Reading will be virtually impossible, but moving around will remain safe – with care!

Ophthalmic examination

This is a vital examination for any serious eye disease in order that the basic cause for the difficulty with seeing may be diagnosed. Much can be learned from a good sighting of the retina. Diseases ranging from diabetic retinopathy (changes in the retina caused by the generalized disease of diabetes, which is an upset in the proper metabolism of sugar), through glaucoma to macular degeneration, to name but a few, can be detected. (The ophthalmic picture of some of the conditions will be described in a following chapter when other visual problems are discussed.)

The examination will take place in a darkened room so there are no other brightly lit images to distract either patient or examiner. In order to obtain a good view of the back of the eye you will be asked to fix your vision on a certain object or small light in the room at a distance, and to keep your eye as still as possible. This is not an entirely easy thing to do, as it is all too tempting to

- try to see what is happening;
- to move away from the bright light of the ophthalmoscope.

It is important, though, to try and cooperate as much as possible, as a much more informative view can be obtained with a 'still' eye.

Some people query whether shining a bright light into the eye is damaging in any way, but be reassured that in no way does this do any harm at all, despite its being a not altogether comfortable experience.

First of all the ophthalmoscope is shone onto the surface of the eye. A 'red reflex' is thus obtained. This shows that the retina is being lit up by the light from the ophthalmoscope. On occasions this red reflex is diminished. This is due to some opacity between the cornea and the retina. The most common cause for this is a cataract in the lens of the eye. This obviously diminishes the amount of information that can be obtained by ophthalmic examination, and so can cause added difficulties (further discussion on this in a later chapter).

Again, difficulties can occur if glasses are worn to correct either a severe long or short sight. Under these circumstances it may be necessary to undertake the ophthalmic examination with the usual spectacles in position. It is only if the refractive error is large, however, that this is necessary.

The retina then has to be brought into focus. This is done by changing the focus in the ophthalmoscope. As this is being done a series of small clicks are heard as the ophthalmologist views the depths of the eye until the retina can be seen in detail. Then the specific changes of macular degeneration are obvious, if this is the cause of the visual difficulties being experienced. In the early stages this may only be a slight raising of the tissue in the macular area. If the condition is further advanced, the yellowish deposit is seen if the dry type is present. The wet type (the least common) shows as a darker red area due to the overgrowth of tissue in the deep layers of the retina.

With the retina in full view other aspects of the health of this vital visual area are examined. For example the state of the blood vessels can be checked for other forms of retinal disease (see later in the chapter).

Once the diagnosis has been accurately made and the type of macular degeneration known, any possible treatment and coping strategies can be addressed.

The news that macular degeneration is the cause of the visual problems can be devastating, and particularly so if the commonest (the dry type) is present. While there is no specific treatment possible at the moment it is important that

- it is explained that complete blindness will not result. Adequate peripheral vision will remain so that independence is not lost;
- there are many coping strategies available so that much of daily living can be done with reduced vision;
- there are a number of societies, with much understanding and help, in existence. Meeting up with other people with similar problems can do much to relieve the feelings of isolation that can be such a part of the news of macular degeneration;
- research is ongoing to find both methods of helping to reduce the difficulties associated with macular degeneration as well as ways of preventing the condition occurring in the first place.

Following diagnosis and introduction to relevant local and national societies the progress of the disease needs to be monitored on a regular basis as well as encouragement given in dealing with the restrictions which will be put on the sufferer. If the wet type is present, further investigation is needed to determine if laser treatment will be helpful.

Fluorescent angiography can be helpful under these conditions. For this test a specific dye is injected into a vein in the arm. This passes through the blood system including the blood vessels in the retina. In this way an informative map of the blood vessels can be seen, including the overgrowth in the deep layers of the retina. (This test is not necessary or suitable for everyone with macular degeneration. Only people with the wet type will be selected as laser treatment is effective only for some people with this type. It is of no value at all in the dry type of the disease. So if this specific test is not suggested to everyone, remember there are very good reasons for not performing it.)

There are a few effects of this injection of dye into the blood system. Occasionally there may be a faint yellowish discolouration of the skin for a day or two afterwards, but this will fade without trace. Also occasionally there may be a mild feeling of nausea at the time of the examination. Again this will not persist for long.

Electrical tests are becoming available. These are of more help in young people with the inherited form of macular degeneration – Stargardt's disease or juvenile macular dystrophy.

A field of vision test defines the area of peripheral vision. It can either be done initially at the first examination or at a later time during the follow-up period. It is also useful to do the test at differing periods of time to follow any progression of the disease. And again it can be helpful to know just what side or peripheral vision each individual has, so that advice on strategies to use the remaining vision to the best advantage can be given.

For this test the patient's gaze must be fixed on a central point in a screen in a darkened room. At intervals a light of varying intensity is shone at the outer edges of vision. When this is seen – still with the eye fixed on the central point – a buzzer is pressed to indicate it is visible at the periphery. In this way a map of what can actually be seen is produced by a computer. Again this does require some degree of concentration to fix and hold one's gaze on the central spot of light. It is all too tempting to look towards the other spots of light being shown.

Field of vision tests are useful in other forms of eye disease – glaucoma, for example.

Serial readings are important in any eye disease where field of vision tests are useful in assessing the progress or otherwise of the specific disease.

These are the tests commonly performed to determine whether or not age-related macular degeneration is the cause of the visual difficulties, and also to find out which type is present.

The next chapter will give brief descriptions of other common eye diseases which can affect the older age group and how they can be treated.

Summary

- A brief history of any family member with visual difficulties will be taken, but this is of less importance than for diseases in other parts of the body.
- A routine check of distance and near vision will be done.
- Examination of the retina with an ophthalmoscope is an important part of the diagnosis.
- Fluorescent angiography is only necessary for a few specialized types of macular degeneration.
- Field of vision tests at regular intervals will assess progress or otherwise of the disease.

6
Further visual problems

This chapter describes briefly a number of other common eye diseases which can affect the older generation, as does AMD. All these conditions result in loss of, or difficulty with, vision.

The eye is a marvellously constructed organ which does, on occasion, become unable to work with 100-per-cent efficiency. Regretfully, as we have already seen in the case of macular degeneration, this does occur more frequently during the later stages of life. There are, however, a number of other entirely different causes that give rise to visual problems. Some are connected with disease in other parts of the body, the visual difficulty being just one part of the symptomatology of the generalized disease. Diabetes is a good example of this – diabetic retinopathy being the part of the condition that affects the eyes.

There are some eye conditions which affect the eyes only – cataracts being an example of this. Yet others, such as one specific type of glaucoma, can, on occasions, give rise to generalized bodily illness.

While there are many other conditions affecting the eye these three are among the most common in the older age group. It is interesting to compare and contrast the signs and symptoms of these other diseases with AMD.

Diabetic retinopathy

Diabetes, or diabetes mellitus to give its full name, is a generalized disease in which the metabolism of sugar is upset. Normally the breakdown of sugar and starches in the diet is under the control of a substance, insulin, which is secreted by the pancreas, an organ tucked away behind the stomach.

There are two main type of diabetes. Type 1 most usually occurs in young people, often showing itself in the teenage years or early 20s. In this type there is either no insulin at all produced or such a small amount as to be virtually ineffective. Regular injections of insulin are needed to control this type of diabetes, which is also known as insulin-dependent diabetes mellitus (IDDM).

Type 2 diabetes more frequently occurs in the middle or elderly age group. Here the pancreas produces some insulin, but not in adequate amounts. Alternatively it is thought that for some reason the body is not able to make proper use of the insulin that is secreted. This type is also known as non-insulin dependent diabetes mellitus (NIDDM). Injected insulin is sometimes necessary for Type 2 diabetes, but more usually the blood sugar levels can be controlled by either diet alone or with the help of tablets taken orally.

Diabetes in some degree is thought to affect around one in every 25 people, and does appear to be on the increase in recent years. It is important that treatment is given early to control the condition, and also to be aware of the effects that can occur in other parts of the body – the eye being just one organ that can be affected.

As with macular degeneration it is the retina that can be affected in the diabetic process, but in an entirely different way. It is the blood vessels of the retina that are affected, and three stages of disease can be recognized. The earliest stage is when the blood vessels are only mildly affected, the walls of these vessels being weakened with possible tiny bulges (aneurysms) being seen. Small amounts of blood can then leak. At this stage the central part of vision – the macula – is unaffected. At this time there may be nothing amiss regarding vision, or maybe only some slight difficulty with reading in a poor light. This can, of course, be put down to needing to have spectacles checked.

During the second stage, the area of the macula becomes involved, and it is then that visual problems will be definitely noticed. As with macular degeneration central vision will be affected. Reading and other forms of close work will become difficult, and people's faces and objects straight ahead will be misty and blurred.

The final and most severe stage occurs as the disease progresses. Blood vessels in the retina become blocked and so lose their capacity to supply the retina with necessary nutrients and remove waste products of metabolism adequately. The body reacts to this state of affairs by producing a whole new set of blood vessels. This is known as 'proliferative diabetic retinopathy'. These new blood vessels are, however, not as strong and tenacious as the original vessels. Their walls are weak and tend to leak fluid. They also grow on the inner surface of the retina and into the vitreous fluid which fills the body of the eye. Following the leakage of blood and fluid, scar tissue remains and so effectively destroys the light sensitive cells of the retina. This scar tissue can pull the retinal tissue out of position, so distorting vision, and in the worst cases giving rise to a retinal detachment (see below).

When this stage is reached, normal vision is much at risk. The worst scenario is that a large amount of blood and fluid floods part of the retina. When this occurs vision can be lost immediately and frighteningly. Smaller amounts of leakage will give rise to a patchy loss of vision in differing parts of the visual field.

It is vitally important that early treatment is given for diabetic retinopathy before this final stage is reached, and certainly before vision becomes blurred or with patchy blank spots occurring.

Treatment for diabetic retinopathy is by laser to retain the vision not irretrievably lost due to excessive bleeding. Lasers are intense beams of light which seal off the blood vessels that are leaking. They need to be extremely accurately focused onto the exact position of the vessels that are causing the damage. New blood vessels which are seen to be actively growing can also be treated by more extensive laser treatment.

Laser therapy is a very exact procedure which is done in a specialized ophthalmic unit. It is done in an out-patient clinic, but it is necessary to be prepared for a relatively long visit. Drops are instilled into the eye, both to dilate the pupil, so that the retina can be clearly seen, and also to anaesthetize the surface of the eye. This will take time to become fully effective. To prevent blinking a small contact lens is fitted. Various segments of the eye may need to be treated, so the eye will need to be moved in definite directions throughout the treatment.

Lasers are very bright, and vision may be slightly reduced during the procedure and for a short time after it has been completed. Also tiny black dots may be noticed where some of the blood vessels have been destroyed. (Laser treatment is not painful, but there may be some discomfort, especially after a long session to treat many rogue blood vessels.)

Consequences of proliferative diabetic retinopathy can be life-altering as both peripheral and central vision can be affected in the most severe condition. Following laser treatment, it is mandatory to inform the Driving and Vehicle Licensing Authority (DVLA). Full testing, at a specialized and recognized centre, of visual fields, colour vision and night vision may be necessary to determine whether driving can be undertaken safely.

Diabetes has wide-ranging effects on the body, and perhaps none so noticeable as those on vision, as can be seen by Hugh's story, which puts into full relief the need for early and frequent vision testing as soon as possible after the diagnosis of diabetes has been made.

It must also be remembered that both cataract formation and open-angle glaucoma are more common in people with diabetes. So visual tests of all kinds are vital in this disease, even if the condition is well controlled by diet and tablets without the need for injections of insulin, which is the general case in Type 2 diabetes in older people.

Hugh
Settling into retirement at the age of 61 was no problem for Hugh. House and garden tasks – neglected for years when a

busy working life took up most spare time – had built up. Hugh's other passion, bell-ringing, also had been put on the back burner many times due to a busy work load. But now frequent trips with the church's bell-ringing team were possible – Durham Cathedral one week and a few small churches further south the following week. Driving to these sometimes out-of-the-way destinations was no problem for Hugh.

Health was good until a routine check at the local GP's surgery revealed that Hugh was diabetic.

'But I don't feel ill,' he complained bitterly to his wife Margaret as she firmly put the lid on the tin containing his favourite biscuits.

Within a few months, in spite of strict dietary restrictions, Hugh needed to be prescribed tablets to complement his diet in order to control his sugar metabolism. Later routine checks on blood sugar showed this regime seemed to be holding the condition and all appeared to be well.

Hugh was never one to complain but Margaret noticed that the time of his daily perusal of the newspaper was getting shorter and shorter. He also needed to be near the window or had to switch on a light. 'Print these days isn't what it used to be,' he often grumbled.

'Perhaps you need to go and have your glasses checked,' Margaret tentatively suggested one morning. 'Shall I make an appointment?'

'Maybe, when I've got a minute to spare,' replied Hugh as he set about yet another house improvement task.

But how he wished he had found time to check on his vision a week later. Driving back from the local market town he drew up at a red traffic light.

'Go on, Hugh,' urged Margaret as the car behind gave an impatient toot. 'The lights are green. What's the matter?' she glanced at Hugh. His face was white and he was covering one eye with his hand.

'I – I – can't see, Margaret – nothing at all out of this eye,' and Hugh gestured towards his left eye. 'This – this

41

one's OK, but the other one is covered with a big black splodge.' With a good deal of effort Hugh set the car in motion and drew into the side of the road a few yards ahead.

'Let me drive,' Margaret took control of the situation. 'I think we'll go straight back to the hospital.'

Several hours later they were back at home, Hugh with his feet up and a mug of tea in his hand. 'You were right, Maggie. I should have taken more care – I really have been having difficulty seeing with this eye just lately. Perhaps a visit to the optician would have avoided this.'

The upshot of this worrying event was that Hugh had suffered a retinal haemorrhage due to his diabetes. Some vision returned but over the succeeding weeks laser treatment was done to seal off the leaking blood vessels. This held the condition for a time, but later the diabetic retinopathy spread to the macular region of Hugh's eye, and he could see very little out of this eye.

Checks need to be done – and are being done – to be sure that Hugh's other eye remains as normal as possible. At present he is still able to drive – after stringent tests to be sure he is safe, instigated by the DVLA. Sensibly Hugh restricts his driving to familiar places during daylight hours.

Diabetic retinopathy is an unpleasant condition resulting from the generalized disease of diabetes, and maybe if Hugh had had his vision checked earlier this problem could have been avoided.

Glaucoma

Glaucoma is a common cause of blindness in the world. It most usually occurs in the over-40 age group and increases in incidence until by the age of 80, more than 10 per cent of people suffer from the disease. Certain groups of people are more at risk than normal and these include:

- people who have someone in the immediate family with the disease. (In the UK eye tests are free for anyone who has a first-degree relative (mother, father, etc.) with glaucoma);
- those people who are very short-sighted;
- those people who are diabetic;
- people of Afro-Caribbean origin.

Every routine eye test at the optometrist includes a check for glaucoma.

As with macular degeneration, glaucoma can assert itself subtly – few symptoms in the early stages being noticed. Again there is loss of a specific part of the visual field, and it is important that regular eye tests are done in the older age group to diagnose glaucoma in the early stages.

There are a number of types of glaucoma, the two most common being:

- chronic open angle glaucoma
- acute angle closure glaucoma.

Other more unusual types are connected to other conditions arising in the eye, the glaucoma being secondary to these.

Glaucoma is characterized by:

- a raised pressure inside the eye;
- field of vision defects;
- specific changes seen on examination with the ophthalmoscope.

There is a constant flow of fluid in the eye in order to maintain its shape and function. This is normally kept at a steady pressure by a complex series of secretion and drainage activities throughout the eye. It is when this beautifully organized system becomes blocked that a rise in the pressure inside the eye results – this being known as glaucoma.

Chronic open angle glaucoma is the most common type of glaucoma. This comes on gradually – in fact so gradually that it is not noticed until some damage has been done to vision. As with macular degeneration there is no pain associated with glaucoma, and it is unusual for the sufferer to notice that a certain part of their visual field is missing. Most usually glaucoma of this type is picked up at a routine eye examination – again underlining the need for regular eye checks in the older generation.

Toxometry – in which the pressure inside the eye is checked by a special instrument placed on the surface of the eye – will give information as to the pressure inside the eye. A quick puff of air is all that is felt during this examination.

Once again, it is the examination with the ophthalmoscope which clinches the diagnosis of glaucoma. (Later, field of vision tests will confirm the diagnosis.) In glaucoma the optic disc (a specific area of the retina through which the main blood vessels and nerves course) is altered. The nerve fibres are seen to be atrophied and the blood vessels stretched and bent due to the increased pressure. This will have arisen over many months. The disc itself, normally of a pinkish colour, appears pale and small haemorrhages may be seen in this area. (The optic disc must not be confused with the macula. They are situated side by side a few millimetres apart and fulfil quite different functions.)

Field of vision tests are quite different from those seen in macular degeneration. They arise in specific segments of the peripheral visual field. Often these defects are not noticed by the glaucoma sufferer as the loss of this relatively small part of the visual field can be compensated for over the months in which it occurs. In severe cases, much of the peripheral visual fields are affected. This results in 'tunnel vision', where only central objects can be seen. This is rather like viewing the world through a telescope.

Acute angle closure glaucoma has a different onset altogether. Pain in the eye is an obvious feature, and the eye itself becomes red and vision is blurred. This is due to a rapid rise in pressure in the eye (in sharp contrast to the slow rise in the chronic type of glaucoma). This rise in pressure can be so

44

rapid in onset that, in addition to pain, vomiting is a symptom. Here the normal drainage of fluid is abruptly stopped by the iris sticking to the back of the lens of the eye. This is an unpleasant and dangerous condition which needs immediate medical care.

Occasionally, previous similar attacks can have occurred, but sleep has resolved the problem. This is because during sleep the pupil constricts and so releases the iris from the lens. Nevertheless, if this should happen it is important that medical help is sought to avoid further damage to the eye and a return of the symptoms. Surgery or laser treatment will often be required for this type of acute glaucoma.

Treatment for chronic glaucoma consists of regular instillations of eye drops which usually control the pressure inside the eye. Instillation of eye drops can initially be tricky, and especially so if there is no one around to help in the early learning stages. To instil the drops yourself, first of all be sure that the drops you are using are the correct ones and then check how much has to be instilled. Then tip your head slightly back, pull the lower eyelid down gently and then carefully instil the required amount of prescribed fluid. Close your eye and feel the liquid working its way round your eye. With practice this will really become second nature, however unlikely this may seem at first.

Routine regular checks are needed to ensure that the pressure is remaining at a normal level.

Glaucoma is quite different from macular degeneration – the only common factor being visual difficulties which can come on slowly.

Recent research in Japan has postulated that excessive use of computers for short-sighted people may be a factor in the onset of glaucoma. Further investigations into this are continuing.

Cataracts

Cataracts are the most common cause of blindness in the world today. This condition is usually found in the older age group, although it can occur in younger people, often due to a variety of other conditions. These include diabetes, any previous severe injury to the eye or the long-term necessity for taking steroid drugs for some other illness. Cataracts can also be present at birth in a very small number of babies – these are known as congenital cataracts.

So just what are these cataracts? Cataracts are a clouding of the lens of the eye. Normally the lens is transparent allowing light to pass through so that images from the outside world can fall clearly on the retina. As we have seen the lens also alters in shape due to the action of the ciliary muscles as objects of different focal lengths are visualized. This latter facility will also be lost as the cataract becomes more advanced. In fact some long-sighted people comment that they can read better without their spectacles as their cataracts worsen. This is due to the inability of the faulty lens to adjust as it was able to do before the onset of the cataract formation.

Age is the most important cause of this condition. Around 60 per cent of people between the ages of 50 and 60 years have some degree of cataracts in one or both eyes. By the time 80 years have passed the majority of both men and women will have some degree of cataract formation.

As with macular degeneration, symptoms are slow to arise. These are frequently ignored or put down to the natural ageing process. Reading becomes more difficult. This is particularly so unless lighting in the room is bright enough. While a good light is necessary for reading, direct bright sunlight can be dazzling – the light being reflected off the opacities in the lens. Activities such as driving, recognizing friends across the street and watching television can become difficult. Colour vision also becomes less perfect. Colours appear washed-out or 'muddy'. This is a further reason for older people preferring to wear brightly coloured clothes or choosing more highly patterned, and more distinctively coloured, furnishing fabrics.

On visiting the optometrist, both near and distant vision will be found to be reduced. Care should be taken not to confuse this with a general refractive error due to either long or short sight. But on looking at the eye closely the cataract can be seen as a sepia, or even a white colouration if the cataract is advanced, of the lens. On shining a bright light, as from an ophthalmoscope, onto the eye the normal red reflex can be seen to be absent.

The treatment for cataracts is by surgery. There are no eye drops or other medication that will make any difference. Over the decades the surgical treatment for cataracts has improved out of all recognition. In our grandparents' day the cataract had to 'ripen' (which meant all vision was practically lost) before an operation could be considered. The whole lens was then removed. This meant that gross hypermetropia was the result – i.e. extreme long-sighted vision. This refractive error had then to be controlled by very thick, heavy lenses.

Nowadays there is no need to wait until the cataract is extensive. Ophthalmic surgeons will operate as soon as the clouding of the lens interferes with daily activities. The operation consists of removing the contents of the lens from its capsule and inserting – through a tiny incision – an artificial lens into the capsule.

A short time before the operation, a routine visit is necessary to check the exact measurements of each individual eye so that the appropriate lens to be inserted can be made. The actual operation is usually performed under a local anaesthetic, so that complete consciousness is maintained throughout.

An hour or so before operation, a series of eye drops are inserted at regular intervals. These are

- to anaesthetize the eye so no pain is felt;
- antibiotic drops to eliminate any infection;
- paralysing drops so the eye remains still during the procedure.

The operation takes around 15 minutes. The surgeon explains what is happening throughout the operation, so you are fully aware of what is being done.

A certain amount of care is needed after any surgical procedure, and cataract surgery is no exception.

- After surgery is completed a pad – or maybe a plastic shield – is placed over the eye. This is not the ordinary type of dressing applied after other types of surgery. It is merely there to prevent the eye being bumped or rubbed. It is advisable to keep this in place for the first night following surgery. It is all too easy to rub an eye when half asleep, and there is a small possibility that this could cause damage.

- Eye drops, of differing types, are necessary for several weeks (up to six weeks) after surgery. It is important that these are instilled regularly. A good idea is to keep a diary of 'which drop when' as the necessary pattern can be difficult to remember. This is especially so if – as can be done – the cataracts on both eyes are operated on with only a few weeks in between. In these circumstances it is possible that different drops are instilled into each eye at different times!

- Heavy lifting or strenuous exercise must be avoided for six weeks or so following the operation. Other normal activities can be undertaken.

- Driving should be avoided for at least a couple of weeks. While vision is much improved almost immediately, it will take a little time to become used to this. It may be found that glasses are no longer necessary after cataract surgery, but each individual will receive advice on this.

- If at all possible, avoid getting anything in your eye. Windy days are a potential hazard for this, so avoid such weather if possible. If anything should enter the eye soon after surgery, it is wise to get it checked out by either your GP or the accident and emergency department at the local hospital.

Cataract surgery is one of the most successful forms of routine surgery. The difference made to vision is often referred to as quite incredible – comment being made most frequently on the richness of the colour of the natural surroundings.

As cataracts are slow to develop, diversity in colour is also slowly lost, and so is not immediately noticeable. But on normal vision being restored, the results are spectacular.

Occasionally laser treatment may be needed in the future if vision again becomes blurred. This is not due to any fault in the new lens that has been inserted, but due to a thickening in the capsule of the lens holding the new lens in place. This laser treatment can be done in an outpatient clinic.

For further details of cataracts, surgery and recovery, *Cataract: What You Need to Know* by Mark Watts (Sheldon, 2005) may be useful.

Detached retina

This condition is worth a quick mention, as it can be associated with one or more of the conditions already described. In a detachment of the retina this vital layer is pulled away from the underlying tissues – the choroid and the sclera. This can be partial, or in the worst scenario, involve much of the retina.

It is by the description of what has actually happened to the sufferer that the diagnosis can be made. It is only when detachment is advanced and involves much of the retina that this becomes most easily visible when viewed with an ophthalmoscope.

At the onset of a retinal detachment, an excess of 'floaters' may be seen. Flashing lights may also be apparent. ('Floaters' are transparent or greyish blobs which are seen floating across the visual field. A small number of these are common and particularly so in short-sighted people.) These effects, however, are not always noticeable and it may be only when there is a marked deterioration in vision that help is sought. At this stage the loss of sight is either due to a large part of the peripheral visual part of the retina being affected or due to the macular region being involved.

There are certain predisposing factors which can increase the risk of retinal detachment:

- Short-sighted people are more prone to this condition. Under these circumstances the retina is thinner than usual and so is more easily detached.

- Diabetic people, who have some scarring of the retina, are also predisposed to a detachment.
- Any injury to the eye can precipitate a detachment.
- Treatment is either with lasers if the detachment is small or by surgery to seal the retina back in place and to drain any fluid from the underlying tissue if there is a larger detachment.

Summary

Details of other conditions that can affect vision:

- diabetic retinopathy;
- glaucoma;
- cataracts;
- detached retina.

7

Coping with the diagnosis of age-related macular degeneration

When anyone is told they have AMD, this news can be received in one of two ways depending on whether or not the sufferer has ever heard of the condition. If they have no idea at all and have never heard macular degeneration mentioned, the news may not seem too bad, and especially so if they are told that total blindness will not occur.

Under these circumstances it is wise to ask for more information as to what is actually meant by macular degeneration: Why does it occur? How much sight will be lost? Will the other eye be affected? Can an independent life be maintained? Is there any treatment? to mention just a few of the questions that need to be asked.

Other people may have heard of AMD, or may even know someone, or have a relative, with the condition. Depending on the severity of the disease in the friend or relative the shock of receiving the same diagnosis will be different. It is still important, however, to ask for first-hand knowledge of the disease. Second-hand news is always suspect and each person with AMD will notice and have slightly different effects.

All of the above queries, and probably many others, will need answers from someone knowledgeable on the subject. The optometrist or ophthalmologist are the best people from whom to gain information. Also much information can be acquired from the societies specializing in visual problems.

So, now you have all the information you can possibly absorb at one sitting, and you are home, mulling over the news. This can be truly devastating, and especially so if you had thought just a change of spectacles was all that was needed to restore your failing vision to normal. What to do now? How to begin to cope with the new form your life seems to be taking?

There are a number of ways in which you can begin to dismiss the initial feelings of despair. None of them at first appears easy, but they will need to be faced over the next few weeks and months.

Take stock

To fully understand the position in which you now find yourself, it is important to be as knowledgeable as possible about your visual state. Many questions need to be asked, such as: What has actually happened? How will it progress?

First of all get as much information as possible about your particular type of AMD. Once all the factors which refer to you especially are known, you will feel a certain amount of relief. There is nothing so worrying as getting only part of the picture. Imagination is a powerful process, and very often creates situations far worse than the truth.

Information about macular degeneration can be gained in a number of ways:

- *Your optometrist.* Even if it means making an extra appointment just to clear up some points of possible misunderstanding this will be well worth while. The possible progress of the disease can be explained together with the particular stage at which you find yourself at the present time. Along with this, comes ways of reducing the disability which will be the inevitable conclusion of a diagnosis of AMD.
- *Societies and self-help groups.* These include the Royal National Institute for the Blind (RNIB) and the Macular Disease Society, details of which can be found at the end of this book. Joining a society will also provide extra information regarding available help, plus the fellowship of people in a similar position to yourself. For example the Macular Disease Society publishes a regular journal called *Side View.* Information and ideas are all to be found

52

in this publication. This journal is also available on audio-cassette.

- *The radio*. In the UK, the BBC has a weekly 20-minute programme especially for people with visual problems. This is called 'In Touch' and is broadcast on Radio 4 in the evening on one day of the week at present (check your local listings). Different topics are discussed and even if they are not applicable to your particular situation, it may be of interest to know what is going on in the field of visual problems.
- *Meeting other people with macular degeneration*. As well as gaining helpful information, there is real value in sharing worries and ways of coping with someone who knows exactly what you are talking about.

Think positively

It is always a good policy to try and think positively when in a situation such as the one in which you may find yourself after receiving any difficult diagnosis. Remember you are not alone in your distress. There are many, many other people in the same state as you are – as is evidenced by the statistics of AMD. As well as obtaining information from other people, positive help can be gained by observing just how well they, who are probably a little further along the road than you, are coping with the difficulties that at present may seem insurmountable to you.

Remember too that AMD is not a painful disease. People with conditions such as rheumatoid arthritis and – in the realms of visual conditions – glaucoma can suffer a good deal of pain. This is in addition to restrictions in daily living. There is little so debilitating as constant pain. Much can be done, of course, to relieve chronic severe pain, but at least this is one disability with which someone with AMD will not have to contend.

Remember as well that with a diagnosis of AMD total blindness will not result. So, although adaptations to daily tasks will have to be made, independence will not be totally lost. Getting around your own home and around other familiar places will be quite possible with a little practice and care.

Tell friends and relatives about your diagnosis of AMD. It is nothing of which to be ashamed. It is incredible how reluctant many people are to inform friends of their disabilities – as if it were their fault that illness of one kind or another has struck. The only problem with AMD is that it is an age-related condition. No one can alter the fact that the years pursue their relentless course. This afflicts us all. A good idea when telling friends of the diagnosis is to give a brief outline of what you have already learned about the condition. In this way, other people too will be aware of the facts, such as AMD is not painful and that total blindness does not result, for example.

Do not be backward in accepting offers of help that will doubtless be forthcoming, and inform friends of the specific difficulties you are experiencing. Many people on learning of someone else's disease will say, 'Anything I can do to help' without really knowing what they can do to help. So tell them!

It is always advisable to give as full an account as possible of just what is amiss with your vision. It is surprising how unintentionally unkind some people can be, say, by suggesting you probably just need a change of glasses. Remember to the outside world your eyes look the same as they always have. It is only you who is aware that seeing is a problem. So do explain your difficulties to friends.

Remember too to sort out in your own mind just what actions and tasks are most difficult. Get help with these and not the tasks you can do for yourself with a little practice.

Think ahead

After receiving the initial diagnosis it can be all too easy to be confused as to what you can manage to do and what will be difficult, or impossible. Wait a little while before you alter completely your lifestyle and immediate surroundings.

It may be a good idea to write down the tasks and living arrangements that you think may prove to be difficult in the future, or which perhaps you are finding less than easy at the present time.

First of all consider your home, be it a house, a flat or a bungalow. No need, as yet, to think of moving unless, of course, this has already been on the cards. There are many minor adaptations that can be done to ensure you can continue to live in your present accommodation easily and safely. This is important and especially so if you are attached to your home and have lived there for many years. Friends nearby are an added bonus and moving away will probably mean that this source of help and companionship will be not so easy to continue. (One friend of mine who lived in a dormer bungalow always went upstairs to bed. The bedroom and en-suite bathroom had spectacular views over the Scottish countryside. But she and her husband decided, quite early on after the diagnosis of AMD, that the spiral staircase to this hideaway was not a good idea! So they now use the downstairs bedroom routinely and send their guests upstairs. Relatively small adjustments such as this mean that familiar places need not be entirely abandoned.)

While you are still thinking of where best to live, the convenience of shopping for everyday needs has to be considered carefully. Remember that vision will not be totally lost, so getting around familiar streets, where everyone is known and helpful, will be possible with care. Perhaps too, it will be a good idea to make enquiries about deliveries of routine foods. Again this will be easier to organize if living in a familiar place. Consider also doing a 'big food shop' once a week (if you are not already doing so). Also, why not organize a local taxi firm to take and fetch you to do this? This will also obviate the need to carry heavy volumes of everyday goods, which is always a disadvantage if public transport is used.

Local activities associated with societies, churches and other organizations already belonged to will be a further advantage to staying put. Helpful friends will be available to escort you to meetings, services and other activities – all part of staying active and mobile. Perhaps now will be the time to start something new. For example, why not join a music group if you are even only vaguely interested in music, but have never had time to pursue further this possible interest?

Reading groups are also becoming very popular. Many books are available on audio tape, so failing vision will not be a problem here. Having listened to the book, joining in the subsequent discussion will be quite possible. New friends can be made this way as well as gaining different interests.

As one ages there is always the thought that perhaps it would be wise to move nearer to family members. This can be a difficult decision to make at any time and not to be undertaken lightly. Children have their own lives to lead, and these do seem to be obsessively frantic these days. Also demands of work may force them to move house at relatively frequent intervals. Most young people seem to spend very long days at work, with also perhaps a good deal of travelling involved as well, so that their company would not be available to you during the day. So do think carefully before uprooting yourself from all your long-term friends and neighbours – after all they are ageing too and may not be able to visit so easily in the future.

Living accommodation can be a problem as one gets older and particularly so if either spouse has died. Each circumstance is different but it is important that far-reaching decisions are not rushed, particularly if there has been a bereavement. Take time to consider all possibilities before making any major decisions. It is not easy to move back again if a precipitate move has been made. Talking over options with family and friends will make matters clearer, but do remember it must be you who is happy with any decisions that are made.

Before making any major steps towards moving house, think about how your current home may be adapted to your present conditions. Further consideration of this will be made in the next chapter. Adaptations will obviously depend on the degree of your disability and may, of course, have to change over the succeeding years. Keeping in touch with your optometrist and asking for an honest opinion as to the progress, or otherwise, of your disease will help in the decision-making process.

Finally, learn how to maximize the sight you do have. Find out about low-vision aids – more later – and how to use your peripheral vision to full advantage. Find the whereabouts of low-vision clinics in your locality. Your optometrist will be able to assist you in this. There are many ways in which remaining sight can be used which you may not have thought possible in the early days following your diagnosis.

Summary

- Find out all you can about your condition.
- Take stock of the situation in which you find yourself.
- Think positively.
- Think ahead.
- Do not rush any decisions about your living accommodation.
- Maximize your remaining sight.

8
Practical help

There are many aspects of daily living that need to be considered when vision is limited. These range from routine tasks around the house, through visits outside the home to the social aspects of day-to-day communication with other people. All these need to be looked at separately to make life less burdensome and also to retain independence. Advice from a low-vision clinic is of enormous help. Here advice is given on how best to cope with differing situations, and on specific aids tailored to each individual's needs. Even if such facilities are not readily available in your immediate area, it is well worthwhile making time – and the effort involved – to visit such a place at least once. Much can be learned from just one visit, and possible arrangements can be made for future needs. The RNIB can give information as to where to find the nearest low-vision clinic to your address. (Postal address and contact information for the RNIB are at the end of this book.)

What happens at a low-vision clinic?

First of all, an assessment is made of the actual degree of visual loss, which will be slightly different for each individual. Also at this time it is important to consider the circumstances in which you are living. Have you a partner who can assist with daily tasks? Or are you living alone? Are there any relatives or friends who can help out on a regular basis? The answers to these, and many other questions, will all add up to the best advice being given on the optimum equipment and training to suit each person.

There are a multitude of aids available – each suited to individual needs. It will take time and effort to make the best possible use of the equipment recommended. Some clinics offer facilities for borrowing pieces of equipment so they can

59

be tried at home before an actual purchase is made. Remember that things may seem more difficult at home on your own instead of being in an environment where help is readily available.

Remember the aim is to make the maximum use of remaining sight so that as much independence as possible can be maintained.

As will be seen as each aspect of living is examined more closely, light, magnification and contrast all play key parts. These will vary, of course, according to the various tasks being undertaken, but it is a good idea to keep these three standbys in mind while thinking about how best to cope with each new situation that arises as you become accustomed to reduced vision.

Light

It may seem an obvious statement, but good lighting is vital for anyone with any degree of visual difficulty. This applies to people with presbyopia and cataract formation (to mention just two other causes of less than perfect vision) as well as macular degeneration sufferers. Those of us who are fortunate enough to have light available at the touch of a switch no longer need to rely on the daylight hours to perform necessary tasks – although natural light is probably preferable in most cases. Anyone will comment on how much better is natural light than artificial light for doing any close work. Nevertheless electric light has revolutionized working practices of all kinds over the decades.

An exception to the benefits of natural light is the glare that can arise from bright sunlight. This can be a particular problem for people with macular degeneration. As we have already seen, the effects of too bright sunlight can be ameliorated by sunglasses or a wide-brimmed hat. While indoors move as far as possible into a position of good light, but out of direct sunlight. As the weeks go by the most suitable position in the room for close work will become apparent.

Sunlight can also be uncomfortable for people with

advancing cataracts, as the light seems to reflect off the opaque lens, giving the impression of everything being covered in bright points of light.

To make the most of the natural light during the day when at home, a few tips are worth remembering – perhaps obvious, but which can be overlooked.

Always sit near a window if possible when working on any task that requires as much visual acuity as possible. Move furniture around so that tables and chairs gain most from the light coming through the windows. If possible working surfaces in the kitchen should also be as near as possible to the source of light, but again out of direct sunlight.

Curtains need to be drawn back as far as is reasonably possible so as not to inhibit the amount of available light. Net curtains also need to be drawn back as far as possible when working. Perhaps remove them altogether except when they are really necessary for privacy. It is surprising how much light these seemingly flimsy curtains exclude.

Windows also need to be kept as clean as possible. Every speck of dirt can reduce vital light rays. This also applies to spectacles if they are worn. The amount of light lost by spotted glasses is quite amazing. Similarly glasses need to be kept free from scratch marks. To ensure this, keep them in appropriate cases when they are not in use – and never, never put them face down on any rough surface. If they should get scratched, visit your optician and obtain a replacement lens. This will be well worth any cost involved.

Adequate and suitable artificial light on dark evenings is also important. Fluorescent lights are better for vision than soft-shaded lamps – no shadowy corners to detract from the main source of light. Perhaps not such an attractive form of lighting but for any degree of close work invaluable.

For reading, writing or any other close work a one-point source is ideal, such as an angle-poise lamp. This can be adjusted to fall exactly on the position most needed for the best illumination. To avoid glare, for example from a sheet of white paper as on a page of a book, it is preferable to have the light coming from the side. A light beside you on a table will probably afford better illumination than one overhead. Trial and error will decide which is best for each individual. Clip-on spot lights are also available to illuminate specific areas. These can be used for desks where reading or writing is done as well as in the kitchen when food is prepared. (While on the subject of glare in general whether inside the house or out and about, tinted lenses in glasses can be helpful. This needs to be discussed with your optometrist who will be able to give advice in individual circumstances.)

It is a good plan to check on the general lighting around the house. Particular reference needs to be made to good lighting at both the bottom and top of the stairs, and also at any changes in levels there may be around the house, such as changes from carpeting to wood floors. Front and back doors will probably be difficult to illuminate fully, but with long-term familiarity with these openings tripping will be less likely. All parts of the home will be familiar, of course, but in the early days of failing vision it is wise to highlight potential problem areas.

All these aspects of lighting can be adjusted in your own home. A visit to family or friends, however, can produce traps for the unwary by way of steps, stairs, edges of rugs for example. It is incredible how easy it is to trip over the edge of a rug if vision is limited. People with full vision are often unaware of this danger, and other potential hazards. Do not be backward in asking about any possible difficulty. People are only too willing to give help and/or explanation if asked.

Magnification

In contrast to the need for good lighting in every situation, the amount and type of magnification needed will vary for each different activity. For example, the type of magnification needed for close indoor activities such as reading, writing, sewing or any other task needing fine vision will be different from that needed for outdoor activities. In these latter conditions, reading bus numbers, railway and airline details or large notices in shopping precincts will need different low-vision aids from those required at home. Yet again, watching television at a comfortable distance from the screen, the necessary magnification will be different.

There are many different low-vision aids to deal with all these circumstances. These include magnifiers that are hand-held. These will be useful when shopping, so details and prices of products can be scanned. These sorts of magnifiers are also useful around the house for seeing details on cookers, central heating settings, washing machines and other pieces of household equipment. Also available are illuminated hand-held magnifiers – useful in the darker recesses of some shops.

Most of these hand-held devices have a fixed focus, and so need to be held close to the surface to be read. Again practice in their use will make the help they can give that much greater. Practically all are small enough to be carried in a pocket or handbag with very little trouble.

Still in the category of hand-held magnifiers are the adjustable tiny telescopes that are useful when visualizing street signs and notices. These are also of value in cinemas, theatres and also at home when watching television. Small binoculars are also available if both eyes are affected by AMD. Far better to sit at a comfortable distance in a favourite chair than sit in discomfort nearer the screen.

Magnifiers on an adjustable stand are of use around the house and when doing static tasks such as sewing, jigsaw puzzles as well as other everyday jobs such as changing electric plugs – with care, of course! The main advantage of this type of magnification is that both hands are free to perform the task in hand. (The hand-held variety must of necessity limit the type and amount of fine tasks that can be done.) As well as being able to adjust the stands of these devices, some have extending arms. These are useful in the ability they give to extend the distance between object and eye.

The 'Eezee Reader' is a device useful for reading recipes,

labels or instructions (often printed in minute type anyway) on pieces of equipment. This device needs to be connected to a television and an electric socket. It is held in the hand and moved across the reading matter. The typed print will then appear in much enlarged text on the television screen. The one minor disadvantage is that colour is not reproduced so everything, including pictures, appear in black and white.

The 'Horizon TV Reader' is a hand-held camera which plugs into an ordinary television set. As the page is scanned the text will appear enlarged.

Closed circuit television (CCTV) is useful for those people who are computer literate and/or those who need to use a computer for work or some specific leisure activity. Not for everyone perhaps, as this equipment is expensive unless put to good everyday use, but worth considering. Maybe a whole new world will open up when a computer is added to the household!

All these types of magnification may seem excessively daunting at first, and difficult to use with any degree of comfort. This is why it is important that access to a low-vision clinic is helpful. Here all the available aids can be tried out and advice given as to which will be most suitable for each individual's lifestyle. For example, the small binoculars that some people find of value for watching television will not be on the shopping list for someone who has no interest in this form of home entertainment. Again the person who has no need or interest in computing will have no need for CCTV.

These pieces of equipment are available through social services, hospital eye clinics and some specialist opticians. The RNIB or Partially Sighted Society also supply catalogues from which equipment can be bought by mail order. (Addresses are at the end of this book.)

Contrast

This may seem an odd heading to be included alongside the more obvious aspects such as light and magnification. But as you come to terms with restricted vision, it will be obvious why contrast in colour between objects will do much to help everyday living. A few examples include:

Black, or other dark-coloured, felt-tip pens on white paper when making notes of any kind – shopping lists, for example. It is also especially useful to keep these near the telephone so that messages can be taken down and more easily read back again.

Liquids, too, need to be contrasted. For example, brown tea in a brown cup or mug will do nothing to help you know when, or if, the container is full, half-full or empty. By contrast tea in a white vessel will be far more likely to be seen. Similarly white lemonade or other pale liquids will be more readily seen in a dark container than in a glass.

Again, white plates on a white surface can cause difficulties in visualizing the edge of the plate, so food can inadvertently be pushed onto the white table covering. Coloured borders on plates or dishes or a complete contrasting colour to the underlying surface can be much easier to cope with.

Wearing contrasting colours in clothing can be difficult especially as colour vision can be muted with AMD. Advice from relatives or friends can be valuable here. Wearing one-colour outfits may be safer, as long as the different tones of colour – so readily available these days – do not clash. Time spent on a periodic review of your wardrobe can be invaluable. Putting matching, or colour co-ordinated clothes together in the wardrobe can be helpful so that when in a hurry the most suitable outfit is reached, in the knowledge that it will match. Bright bold colours are obviously easier to deal with than soft muted shades. Blue is a particularly difficult colour to visualize as is the difference – previously mentioned – between navy blue and black.

Finally, on general practical hints, is the need to know exactly where everyday objects are kept. To quote one of our grandparents' maxims: 'A place for everything and everything in its place' may be irritating but it is definitely helpful for people with restricted vision. Knowing the bread knife will always be found on the right-hand side of the top kitchen drawer will save much searching and frustration – as well as perhaps an unfortunate injury. Other people living in the house will also need to be reminded to be sure to put things back in their original position.

It is a good idea to do a check at the end of the day to be sure that things in everyday use are all in their proper place. Early morning hiccups about finding things before starting the day can be avoided.

It is also important that objects should not be left lying in exposed places where they can be tripped over easily. Special care in this context needs to be taken when, for example, grandchildren or young nieces and nephews are visiting.

These tidy habits are obviously only of use in one's own home. Visits to family or friends can produce hazards, and especially so where there are children involved. But do not be backward in asking for help when visiting. Family and/or friends will be only too happy to be made aware of the potential hazards that may be around and so reduce as far as possible any risk of injury.

Summary

- Light, magnification and contrast are the three mainstays for easier living.
- Make family and friends aware of potential hazards in their homes.
- Ask for help.
- Keep everything as tidy as possible.

9
Possible areas of difficulty

Certain areas of the house do present extra problems to people with restricted vision. General living areas do have their hazards, but it is the kitchen, bathroom and stairs that need extra care.

Returning to the everyday living rooms in a house for a moment it may seem obvious to avoid rugs raised in height from a wooden floor or carpet. It is all too easy to forget where they have been placed and so trip over them. In a similar way, rugs on polished floors are a hazard to anyone by slipping but especially so to visually restricted people. Remember that a panoramic view of a room is possible for people with macular degeneration. It is when focus is brought to bear on objects within the central visual range that the offending hazard becomes invisible – more on this later.

Perhaps in the review of general living accommodation it would be better to avoid rugs and mats altogether at home.

Still in the general living area, heating from electric, gas or open fires needs to be approached with care. Especially dangerous can be the objects left on the mantelpiece over the source of heat. Stretching over the fire to secure something needs to be approached with caution. Better to remove all such objects to a less dangerous place. This practice does, of course, apply to anyone, with or without a visual handicap. Children can be especially at risk, unless firmly prevented from reaching over a fire to obtain something from the mantelpiece. But as with other everyday hazards, extra care does need to be taken if visually restricted.

Pets, too, can create hazards. Balls and doggie toys left lying around on the floor can be tripped over, as well as the sleeping pets themselves. Dogs and cats should, if possible, be encouraged to use their own beds/baskets for dozing – but a warm fireside can be extremely tempting. Also domestic animals are not known for their abilities to put their toys in a safe place. It is not necessary to avoid keeping pets. On the contrary they can be a great source of comfort and companionship for anyone whose daily activities are restricted for whatever reason – just a little extra care is necessary.

Still on the subject of pets – arrangements need to be made to take a dog out for a daily walk, for example. Perhaps an opportunity to go along with the 'dog-walker' on a welcoming sunny day? Or perhaps it may be possible to walk alone on a well-known route?

Cats are probably less of a liability than dogs. Their 'exercise' can be obtained just by opening a door – or putting in a cat flap if one does not already exist. But do not discount having a pet altogether. They really are great company.

Kitchen

The kitchen is a potentially dangerous place for both the young and those of more mature years, and especially if there is also an added visual handicap. Here again, it is vital that saucepans, kettles and other everyday equipment are all kept ready to hand and not moved from their accustomed places. This applies also to everyday items such as spoons, whisks, and tin-openers, which are kept in cupboards and drawers. This habit of general tidiness will come as second nature to those people who have been used to organizing their lives in this way. But we are all different, and other people may have to make a deliberate effort to keep articles used every day in certain well-remembered places.

The rest of the family also need to be aware when visiting that they too need to be meticulous in returning articles to their agreed places. If this is not done it may only become apparent after the family have returned home – and you find yourself searching for that vital piece of equipment.

Much kitchen equipment is frequently kept in drawers. Here there can be confusion however carefully equipment is put away. An alternative idea is to hang such everyday tools on a board kept in a convenient position. Magnetic boards are obtainable which can be invaluable for keeping objects such as knives, scissors and other potentially dangerous equipment. Other larger objects such as whisks, wooden spoons, tin-openers – the list is endless and unique to each person's kitchen – can also be hung in their own specific positions.

The markings on cookers, washing machines and other electrical goods can be a problem as central vision is of importance in reading the dials to set the right temperature, speed and programme. The most frequently used settings can be marked boldly with brightly coloured stickers, marking pens or 'bumps' – raised stickers which can be easily felt. Different types of these can be purchased from the RNIB, the Partially Sighted Society or loaned initially from a low-vision clinic.

Gas cookers can present a hazard when the gas is being lit. To avoid burns from this activity, settle the saucepan firmly on the cooker *before* lighting the gas. In this way the danger of a sudden upsurge of flame can be prevented. Electric cookers have a different form of hazard. It can be all too easy not to turn off fully the heat source. This will leave the electric ring slightly hot until the cooker is used again – a source of burnt fingers if the ring is accidentally touched.

A recent article in *Side View*, the magazine of the Macular Degeneration Society, entitled 'Energy Watch' informed readers that partially sighted people can register on the Priority Services register. This will make available certain services, such as an annual safety check if all adults in the house have a visual or other handicap. For further details the appropriate gas or electricity supplier should be contacted. *Side View* has many helpful ideas and practical help tips such as the above.

On the cooking theme, a microwave is a helpful piece of kitchen equipment. It will, of course, be necessary to be conversant with the settings on your specific machine – here again, coloured stickers can be of use. Advantages are that, provided the settings are correct, burnt saucepans are a thing of the past. Washing up is saved as well as electricity. Remember, however, to take care when removing cooked food from a microwave. While the containers themselves are not hot, the contents are!

Storage of food stuffs can present problems in discerning which substance of similar texture is being found. Keeping similar food stuffs, such as rice, flour, desiccated coconut, in different shaped, and/or different highly coloured, containers will prevent difficulties in distinguishing between sugar and flour, for example, or loose tea and coffee granules.

As the days go by, each individual person will find ways of coping with daily tasks specific to themselves. Talking about various strategies at a low-vision clinic or with other members of a visually impaired society can be very helpful. It is amazing how inventive many people can be with excellent ideas to be shared. A simple shared idea can lead on to other ways of coping in the kitchen.

It may be necessary to adopt ways of preparing food differently from those which have been practised before. For example, and particularly in the early days after diagnosis, it can be helpful to use some commercially prepared meals and/ or ready-washed and prepared vegetables and salads. This can be especially helpful if living alone with no one to check that vegetables, for example, are adequately prepared. Do not think of this as lazy or habit-forming. Just a sensible adaptation – and maybe only temporary – to a different lifestyle.

Bathroom

The bathroom can also present specific hazards when vision is less than perfect. For example, the level of the water in the bath needs to be checked by hand to prevent overflow, and alternatively, of course, only an ankle-deep amount. Also it is important to check the temperature of the water if it is impossible to visualize the rate at which the water is running into the bath. Showers can be a good alternative to baths, as there is no chance of overflow.

As with other rooms in the house, towels, soap, etc. need to be kept in specific places so that they may easily be found. Grab rails too can be useful when getting out of the bath. Also do take note of the advertised different types of baths and showers available these days for older people. For example, showers with seats can be especially helpful for those with visual difficulties.

Still in the bathroom, make sure that toilet rolls are renewed at regular intervals or at least have replacements in a handy position. And especially so if living alone with no one near to call in an emergency!

Stairs

If living accommodation is on more than one floor, stairs can have their difficulties. Here it is especially vital to have good lighting, particularly at the top and the bottom of the stairs. A good idea is to count stairs as they are ascended or descended. If in a hurry it can be easy to miss out on one stair – even if the number is very well known. With restricted vision, missing a step could result in an injury. A hand rail or banister can also be helpful to hold on to and so reduce risks of tripping.

It is also worth rethinking living accommodation so that stairs can be avoided altogether if at all possible. If moving to a flat or bungalow is not practicable, perhaps living entirely on one floor is an option. With thought houses can be adapted to one-floor living, by perhaps constructing a downstairs bathroom and toilet. In this way all facilities, bathroom, toilet and kitchen, will be on one level. Perhaps the unused upstairs rooms could be used for family or other visitors? The possibilities are, of course, unique to every individual, but it is worth giving some thought to as living with macular degeneration becomes a practical reality.

But if there is no need for such major upheavals, why not

investigate the possibilities of a stair lift? This could avoid potential difficulties with stairs. Again, this could be something worth considering in the light of your own specific circumstances.

Finally, outside steps in the garden can be usefully highlighted by a white strip painted either on each step or at least on the top and bottom ones.

Summary

- Pets – advantages and disadvantages.
- Areas of potential difficulties – kitchen, bathroom, stairs.
- Coping strategies for these areas.

10

Odds and ends

Reading and writing

Easy reading can be one of the most missed activities once AMD has been confirmed. It has probably been noticed over the preceding months that this everyday activity has become more difficult. Once the cause of the visual problem has been diagnosed and this difficulty explained, now is the time to implement coping strategies. Reading will not be a thing of the past although not the easy delight of before.

Once again the triple aids of light, magnification and contrast will be the best way to continue to enjoy the written word – be it the daily newspaper, favourite magazines or the longer read of a novel. (Perhaps this latter enjoyment may give rise to extra difficulties due to the slower rate of reading that is now necessary. But each individual will find out just what they can or cannot do.)

An angle-poise lamp, situated behind and to one side of the chair is the first aid to easier reading. Try different positions of the lamp to give the best possible light without shadows being cast or too much reflection glaring up from the white paper.

The position of the newspaper, magazine or book can also make a difference to the ease of reading. Rather than laying the paper or magazine flat on a surface try positioning it at around 20 degrees from the horizontal on, for example, an old-fashioned reading stand. This may do much to ease reading and also help you to sit in a more comfortable position.

Trial and error on these two aspects will determine the best position for each individual.

Having the book held closer to the eyes than is usual may also help. This will in no way damage your eyes so do practise holding or resting the reading material at different distances until the maximum comfortable position for you is found.

Large-print books will obviously be an advantage and these can be borrowed from most libraries. The selection may not be as great as the usual supply of books, but requests for definite titles may be possible from other branches, so it is well worthwhile making your specific requests known for large-print books.

'Talking books' are a great source of listening to the written word, and can again be borrowed from libraries. Many books are recorded by well-known actors, and are a great idea for birthday or Christmas presents. There is a large selection of books available in this form, covering many aspects of reading material. Also available are 'talking' newspapers and magazines on audio tape, CD, and as email and internet downloads (see page 97). So make enquiries as to the availability of your own favourite read.

Writing letters or cards can present problems in keeping in a straight line on the paper. Various techniques can be tried using a ruler, and specialized pieces of equipment are available to ease this by writing between thin metal strips. Using a word processor is the other option when needing to communicate in writing. Touch-typing is an advantage here but results will probably need to be checked visually – at first anyway, or unless your touch-typing abilities are meticulous.

While on the subject of writing, difficulties initially may be experienced when shopping and using a credit or debit card. It may prove impossible to use the 'chip and pin' method which most cards now employ. The machine used to punch in the numbers on the credit or debit card may not be clearly visible, so you cannot be certain that the numbers you have punched in are correct. To avoid this problem banks and other credit card organizations issue a card that needs a signature rather than a number to be punched in. These cards are known as 'chip and signature'. Stores taking payment by card will know of this. When the card is inserted into the machine the cashier will be told that a signature is required rather than a number. To obtain such a 'chip and signature' card inform your bank or credit card organization of your difficulty with number punching, and a specialized individual card will be issued.

Shopping

Shopping will not be as easy as before, and strategies to cope with this task will need to be sorted out. As previously mentioned a 'once-a-week' shop for everyday grocery items, for example, may need to be looked into, and especially so if living alone. Perhaps a friend or neighbour who visits supermarkets on a regular basis can be contacted to help with this? Shopping over the Internet is also a possibility if computers are part of your life. Goods then can be delivered without the hassle of travelling, fetching and carrying everyday requirements. If you are fortunate enough to have a younger member of the family who is conversant with computers this can indeed be a bonus and a way of coping with the necessity on a weekly basis.

Shopping for household goods other than food and also for clothes may need the help of a friend or family member. Someone else's opinions on purchases can be useful in this context, and especially perhaps when choosing clothes. Again everyone's circumstances will differ when considering these aspects of living.

Socializing

Social activities of various types will, of necessity, need to be somewhat different from the time before macular degeneration was diagnosed. Much more reliance will be put on auditory stimuli than visual. Theatre performances can still be enjoyed. Perhaps not quite as much as before as the visual impact will be reduced, but nevertheless the spoken word has much to recommend it. Music, too, can be a perhaps greater source of pleasure. The main problem may well be the journey to and from theatres or concert halls, but hopefully friends or group activities can be of help here.

A word about social occasions in general may be of value here. Conversing with previously unknown people can be difficult if their faces cannot be clearly seen. Here, use needs to be made of the remaining, valuable, peripheral vision. This is known as 'eccentric' (away from the centre) vision. A direct central gaze is usually employed when addressing another person, and eccentric vision needs to be learned and practised to become fully useful. It must be remembered, however, that to other people it will appear as if you are looking either over their heads or to a position behind them. This can be disconcerting if the person being spoken to is not aware of your visual problems that are making you seem to be looking in these unusual directions, and misunderstandings may arise from this. They may not even realize it is to them that you are speaking as you appear to be looking elsewhere. It is a good plan to actually articulate the person's name to whom you are proposing to speak before actually starting the conversation. In this way they will be sure it is to them that you are speaking and not to someone else behind them. With familiar people this will, of course, not be necessary. It is, however, a good coping strategy to apply if in the company of strangers who are not aware of your difficulties.

A further potential misunderstanding can occur with someone who is not fully aware of how macular degeneration affects vision. Panoramic scenery can still be enjoyed to a certain extent when suffering from this condition. Peripheral vision plays a good part at looking at a large scene. It is only when focusing on the smaller parts of the scene requiring central vision that difficulties arise. So to someone unaware of the precise problem it may appear that vision is not as severely affected as it is in reality. So again misunderstandings can arise when closer objects need to be visualized. Just one more difficulty in explaining about macular degeneration!

Every person with macular degeneration is affected differently, and this will include the type of circumstances in which they are living. There is one special set of circumstances that can cause extra difficulties. This is when living alone following the loss of a husband or wife – and this, of course, is more likely to happen as age advances. This often occurs just at the time of life when macular degeneration makes its unwelcome presence known. Under these conditions all help possible from family and friends needs to be sought – very necessary after widowhood anyway, but especially so for people with AMD.

One or two special situations come to mind. Neighbours need to be asked to check that the curtains are drawn back each day – or if not to make contact to be sure that all is well. Perhaps drawing back the curtains in the mornings is a small task that has become routine over the years, but one which may be forgotten if vision is dimmed.

Following on from this, neighbours need to be trusted with a key to your house in case help is needed at any time. But do remember not to leave the key in the lock as you close up for the night. If you do so, no one will be able to get in if an emergency should arise.

Registration as partially sighted

In Britain, local authorities hold a register of blind and partially sighted people who live in their area. This registration is entirely voluntary on behalf of the affected people, and there is no pressure at all for such registration. There is, however, help that can be available if registered. For example, an attendance allowance, for visually impaired people over 65 who need help with various everyday activities. A further example is free NHS vision tests. A number of leaflets are available regarding other benefits, obtainable from the RNIB or the Macular Disease Society.

A new system of registration has recently been instituted. Local optometrists are now able to give a referral letter to be sent to the local social services department. Local ophthalmologists will also alert the social services to the problem so that appropriate help can be given. Hopefully this new system will open more doors to aids in general living.

So while it is not mandatory to be registered as partially sighted a recent RNIB survey found that being registered was helpful when applying for various aids and possible financial help in some circumstances.

In Britain also, the recent advent of the Disability Discrimination Act can have advantages for partially sighted people such as, for example, regulations regarding design of, and access to, public transport. Legal problems concerned with disabilities in general can also be dealt with. Further details on all aspects of disability can be found at the Disability Rights Commission (DRC), the address of which is to be found at the end of the book.

Summary

- Coping strategies for reading and writing.
- Social activities.
- Registration as partially sighted.
- Disability Discrimination Act.

11
Diet and exercise

As well as considering ways of coping with AMD – and other visual problems that can occur – we will take a look at general preventative measures that may help prevent the onset of macular degeneration. Many of these measures also help to promote general good health. When looking at 'Risk factors' a number of headings were briefly discussed – diet, smoking and alcohol. The next two chapters look in more depth at these facets of healthy living, together with the general benefits of exercise (even if of necessity limited with AMD) in keeping 'stability', 'strength' and 'suppleness' in as good a condition as possible.

Diet

Probably more has been written about diet, in a variety of contexts, than most other aspects of our daily lives. Diets to lose excess weight are among the most sought after in our current western explosion of obesity. Yet other people need more nutritious diets to gain weight when they are recovering from a vicious bout of infection, or are suffering from the effects of some long-term illness.

Then there are diets for people suffering from disease such as coeliac disease (in which the gluten component found in wheat and some other cereals is the cause of their disease). And people with diabetes – also much on the increase in western society – need to be careful of their diet in which the metabolism of sugar is upset due to lack of, or insufficient amounts of, insulin, a substance secreted by the pancreas.

Also there are diets for vegetarians. There are a number of different types of vegetarians ranging from strict vegans where only vegetables are eaten to less strict where fish and eggs are eaten with just meat being avoided entirely.

All these diets are quite specific to the condition which is being either treated or considered together with, of course, the appropriate medical treatment.

Diets to prevent or restrict the progression of AMD are less specific, and to some extent controversial. Nevertheless it is known that some aspects of diet have an effect on vision.

Vitamins play a part in a good, healthy diet. They are not part of the 'building blocks' of the body, such as are proteins. Neither do they provide energy as do carbohydrates and fats. Rather they regulate enzymatic and other biochemical processes necessary for the proper function and health of the body. Vitamins are substances found in a variety of foods from both animal and vegetable sources.

A number of these substances are necessary for good health, but three are vital for antioxidant processes, as have been previously described. (As a reminder, the body produces substances known as 'free radicals' during the oxygenation processes necessary for life. These free radicals can damage cells in many parts of the body if they are in excess. 'Antioxidants' are the good guys which mop up these free radicals and so help to prevent disease.)

The vitamins concerned in this process are the ACE group – vitamins A, C and E.

Vitamin A is an important member of this group. It is a fat-soluble substance and is vital in the initial part of the production of the 'rods and cones' in the retina, which, as has been seen, are the all-important 'seeing' part of the visual complex. It is estimated that worldwide around 500,000 cases of blindness and poor vision every year in young children are caused by vitamin A deficiency. This blindness is mainly due to the effects on the cornea and conjunctiva (the thin external covering of cells over the whole front of the eye).

The early onset of night-blindness can be a sign of a deficiency of vitamin A and again is especially common in developing countries of the world.

There are two forms of vitamin A, the first being 'retinol', which is preformed vitamin A and is found in animal foods such as liver, kidney, eggs and dairy produce such as whole milk and cheese. The second, beta-carotene, is a substance which is acted upon by a particular enzyme in the intestine to make vitamin A. This beta-carotene is found in large measure in highly coloured fruits and vegetables such as carrots, peppers and cantaloupe melons.

Vitamin A can be stored in the liver – unlike vitamin C (see later) – and so does not need to be replenished on a daily basis. There is no need to take extra vitamin A if a good mixed diet is eaten. Rarely, but still something to be remembered, overdosage of vitamin A can be a problem. This can be suspected if anaemia, mouth ulcers, blurred vision and chapped lips are noticed. But it must be repeated this condition is extremely rare and only to be found if a vast amount of vitamin A is taken in some form – the person who lived only on carrot juice, for example.

Vitamin C (or ascorbic acid) is the second member of the ACE group and is a water-soluble vitamin. It is well known as a preventative of scurvy in sailors in past centuries. These mariners had no access to any fresh fruits or vegetables for long periods of time. When lemons or limes were added to their diet the cases of scurvy disappeared.

This vitamin cannot be stored in the body, so adequate amounts are needed in the diet every day. As well as preventing such diseases as scurvy (virtually unknown today), vitamin C is essential for the repair of bone, cartilage and other connective tissues. This function is especially essential in childhood, but also vital for the continuing repair of these structures throughout life. It is a natural laxative (although the fibre in the fruit will also help to prevent constipation), and also speeds up the healing of wounds, for example, following any surgical procedure.

Vitamin C has also been said to help prevent the common cold, although this has not been scientifically proven. Nevertheless, many people are convinced that extra vitamin C will help to clear a cold more quickly. This vitamin is found in high amounts in citrus fruits, strawberries, green peppers, cauliflower, green vegetables and potatoes (especially just below the skin of these latter vegetables – so cooking new potatoes in their skins, as well as being a delicious way to eat them will increase the amount of vitamin C in the diet).

Vitamin E (or 'tocopherol') is a fat-soluble vitamin, but unlike other fat-soluble vitamins is not stored in the body for any length of time, so a certain amount of this vitamin is needed in the diet every day. Eating a good mixed diet means this should present no problems. One of the main actions of this vitamin is to prevent cell-membrane damage and so it can have an effect on the conditions that affect these building blocks of life.

This vitamin is found in wheatgerm products, broccoli, eggs and butter. Overdosage with this vitamin is practically impossible.

So, while vitamins cannot be said to be directly involved in the prevention of AMD, it can be seen as essential that one's diet contains sufficient amounts of these substances (particularly the ACE grouping) for general good health.

Vitamins have a very specific effect, but it is important to be aware of the need to eat a good general diet to maintain good health. And the maintenance of good general health is vitally necessary if there is any long-term disability, such as AMD.

General principles of an adequate sensible diet include sufficient amounts of the three mainstays of good nutrition – carbohydrates, proteins and fats. There are a multitude of diets advising various proportions of these basic requirements, but it is not the purpose of this book to look at them in any depth. Rather it must be said that a diet containing a good mix of these three basic groups is essential for health. All necessary vitamins and minerals (the latter of which there are many, but all are needed in only very small amounts for health) will be included if food intake is regular and of a wide variety of all kinds of foods – according to taste, of course! Obviously, amounts of food must be adequate, but not of such a quantity as to cause obesity – which is fast becoming the scourge of western society. 'Moderation' should be the watchword in pursuing a healthy diet.

Exercise

Finally, in this chapter on 'preventative measures', remember that exercise can be a potent factor in preventing some of the difficulties encountered with macular degeneration. It may have been noticed initially as AMD became apparent, that one's balance when moving around was affected. As well as the proprioceptive component of balance – the feel of surroundings by different parts of the body, feet on the ground, for example – vision also plays a part in balance. So when this aspect becomes less than perfect, balance can be affected. The automatic reaction to this impaired sense of balance is to cease moving around, and not going out to different places that were previously enjoyed. And the corollary to this is that muscles become weakened due to disuse. This creates a vicious circle in which less and less exercise is taken. Add to this the initial feelings of disorientation and possible giddiness which can be felt as vision becomes diminished, and it can be seen that trips and falls become more likely to occur.

So to reduce the possibility of muscle weakness becoming a further problem, it is important that muscles are kept in as good a working order as possible.

Walking is one of the best exercises possible, using as it does many of the body's muscles. With failing vision, this particular activity can, of course, become more difficult. But a daily walk around a well-known route will do much to maintain muscle strength, if this is at all possible. Perhaps a walk with a friend occasionally would be possible, or maybe there is a rambling association in your locality to which you would be welcome?

Swimming, too, is good exercise. Many muscle groups are put to use in swimming. The great advantage of this form of exercise is that the surrounding water is buoyant. This makes movement easier while still ensuring muscles are usefully activated. (A friend of mine with multiple sclerosis swims regularly. She finds that the movements which are quite impossible for her on 'dry land' are relatively easy to perform in the water.) Even walking in water is beneficial, as muscles need to be exercised harder when pushing against the weight of the surrounding water. Gentle exercise can also be done in this medium. Maybe you could investigate quiet times at your local swimming pool. Again joining a group for exercise in the pool could be a possibility.

A few gentle stretching exercises done on a daily basis will also help mobility and lessen the chances of an unpleasant fall. Simple tricks like standing on one leg will all help to maintain good balance. Take care initially! Remember visual clues on balance will not be as good as they were previously.

This may all seem somewhat irrelevant as you start learning to cope with diminished vision, but do remember that the aim is to live life as fully as possible within the limits of your particular disability. Keeping a healthy lifestyle with a good, adequate diet and a reasonable amount of exercise will do much towards this aim.

Summary

- Factors to be considered in preventative aspects – diet and exercise.
- Possible role of vitamins – ACE vitamins.
- Exercise to maintain balance.

12

A healthy lifestyle

It is as well to remember also that these lifestyle measures will all help to avoid other common conditions such as heart attacks and strokes. Heart attacks and strokes, together with cancers of all kinds are the biggest killers today. Obesity does not help reduce the likelihood of suffering from these conditions. An adequate and sensible diet can do much to reduce the burgeoning – in the western world – incidence of the massive weight gain that afflicts so many of our citizens. This weight excess in turn does have an effect on the incidence of heart attacks.

The heart is a marvellously adapted pump. It is made up of specialized muscle – cardiac muscle – which has to pump, night and day, continuously throughout life at a regular rate of between 60 and 80 beats per minute. Some task!

This pumping action forces blood, carrying oxygen and nutrients, to all parts of the body through the arteries. This includes, of course, all the fatty tissue in the body, much of which lies around many of the internal organs, as well as that visible to us as we look in the mirror. So it is obvious that if there is an excessive amount of fatty tissue in the body, the work of the heart is increased.

In addition to this an excess of specific fatty substances in the diet can contribute to the formation of fatty plaques in the arteries. Cholesterol, in this context, is the most important of these fatty substances. This is further subdivided into two separate components, one harmful and the other not. The high-density lipo-protein – HDL – protects the arteries and so lessens the risk of a heart attack. The low-density lipo-protein – LDL – is the type more likely to form the harmful plaques in the arteries.

So a diet high in HDL foods is recommended in the fight against heart attacks. Much has been written on the most useful diets which include these specific substances, and can be found in any diet book.

As well as pushing its way past excess fat in many parts of the body, the heart has to work harder than ever when fatty plaques narrow the lumen of the arteries. It is when these plaques – known as 'atheroma' – become large enough to block the arteries which supply the heart muscle – the coronary arteries – that a heart attack can result. The coronary arteries themselves are tiny, no larger than a piece of string, so only a small deposit of fatty tissue can cause problems.

So from this viewpoint, diet and exercise are all part of maintaining a healthy heart.

Similarly the incidence of strokes can be minimized by a healthy diet and a modicum of exercise. There are two types of strokes. First, is the type in which there is a blockage of the artery supplying the brain with oxygen and nutrients – in a similar way to heart attacks. Second, a blood vessel in the brain or associated blood vessels can rupture and destroy brain tissue. This latter type of stroke (or cerebral haemorrhage) comes on suddenly and catastrophically in contrast to the relatively slow blockage of an artery as described before. There are, of course, a number of other factors in the incidence of both heart attacks and stroke. These include high blood pressure and stress levels as well as a genetic tendency.

Nevertheless the general factors of healthy diet and exercise do have a bearing. Nothing but good can result from efforts made in these two areas.

Smoking

As mentioned previously in the chapter on 'Risk factors', one piece of research considered that the possibility of age-related macular degeneration (AMD) occurring was twice as likely in people who smoked more than 20 cigarettes a day. Smoking compromises the action of the protective antioxidants so important in destroying the free radicals which can cause harm in many parts of the body.

It is also a well-known fact that cigarette smoking is a potent factor in the onset of both lung disease and heart disease.

Lung disease and smoking

There are two main conditions of the lung connected with smoking. First, smoking is thought to have a direct correlation with COPD (Chronic Obstructive Pulmonary Disease). This term includes such conditions as chronic bronchitis, emphysema and some severe cases of asthma. The habit of smoking is thought to give rise to a low-grade persistent inflammation of the respiratory tract. In addition the ability of antioxidants to do their job may be reduced.

COPD is a relatively common condition causing much illness and death. It may account for over 10 per cent of all admissions to hospitals in England and Wales. This is a sizeable amount of disability which could be largely prevented by giving up smoking.

Much research has been done into the correlation of lung cancer and smoking. Smoking is considered the most important single factor in the incidence of lung cancer. Both the number of cigarettes smoked and their tar content are thought to be implicated. Although lung cancer can occur in non-smokers it is known that the death rate from lung cancer is 40 times greater in smokers than in those people who do not smoke.

In recent years, deaths from lung cancer have dropped slightly in men, while they have risen in women. This may well be due to the difference in smoking habits in the two sexes.

Heart disease and smoking

Smoking can also have an effect on the incidence of heart attacks, and giving up smoking can help to prevent such events occurring. Within six months of giving up the habit of smoking, the risk of a heart attack is significantly lowered.

As a side-line smoking is also thought to compromise the

action of vitamin C, which as has been seen is a factor for good in the prevention of illness, and conditions such as AMD.

So all in all smoking is not a habit to be recommended. It is worrying to note how many young people (and especially young women) are still smoking these days. Much needs to be done, through education and persuasion, to reverse this trend.

Alcohol

Excessive intake of alcohol can often have a deleterious effect on antioxidants, which in turn can exert effects on many parts of the body, including the eye. This effect does not occur with normal, socially acceptable quantities of alcohol. In fact a small amount of alcohol, especially when accompanied by food, can be beneficial in the avoidance of heart problems.

But just what is an acceptable amount of alcohol on a daily basis? Recommended amounts are expressed in 'units'. Each unit is equivalent to:

- one 125 ml glass of wine (4 per cent by volume)
- one small 50 ml glass of fortified wine, e.g. sherry, port
- one single measure of spirits
- one half pint of beer, lager or cider.

There is also a recommended maximum of daily units commensurate with good health:

- 3 to 4 units per day for men
- 2 to 3 units per day for women
- 2 alcohol-free days per week (although if intake is minimal, this need not be adhered to).

Binge drinking, regretfully so prevalent today, is considered to be more harmful than a regular low intake. (Women's bodies tend to break down alcohol more slowly than men's. This is why the recommended daily amount for women is lower – not because of any gender bias!)

So while alcohol intake is relatively low in the risk factors associated with the incidence of AMD, it is as well to keep to the sensible guidelines in order to maintain good health – an important task when affected by any long-term disability.

Keeping a healthy lifestyle is important when a long-term disability such as AMD is present. The above is a very brief discussion of the main points, which can be found in other specialist books.

Summary

- Role of diet in heart disease.
- Role of smoking in lung and heart disease.
- Need to keep alcohol consumption within reasonable limits.

Conclusion: the future

Sometimes the outlook for people with AMD can seem to be only how to learn to live with their disability. Indeed much needs to be done to make life as bearable as possible by learning appropriate coping strategies – and these *will* certainly make life easier to cope with. But it is important to know that there is a good deal of research going on, both into the causes of the disease and also possible treatment.

Genetic research continues in an endeavour to pinpoint any possible genetic background to the disease. There has been some success in teasing out the genetic inheritance in juvenile macular degeneration. It was hoped that this may lead to related insight into AMD, but unfortunately it has only been possible to find a genetic link in a small number of cases of the age-related condition. Further studies are, however, ongoing and will hopefully lead to further clues about the development of AMD.

Also studies are continuing in Europe into possible causes. Increased risk factors have been highlighted – namely smoking, and excessive exposure to high levels of solar radiation as seen in countries where there is bright sunlight for much of the time. Greatly decreased levels of antioxidants are also considered to be a possible contributory factor; so diet is definitely important. It has been suggested that supplements of antioxidants may halt the progress of AMD. Care needs to be taken, however, in taking excess amounts of such supplements. It is far better to be sure to eat a healthy balanced diet throughout life. In this way an adequate amount of antioxidants will be available for the body to cope with a variety of diseases, macular degeneration being just one of these.

So while it may be possible to alter some of the environmental factors, the causation of AMD does remain something of a mystery. The only definite factors are that it is a disease of older people with a strong bias towards women. Other factors are suspected, but no one facet can be highlighted.

Specialized laser treatment has recently become available for certain types of AMD. Here a dye is injected into the arm, which is then taken up by the tiny aberrant blood vessels in the retina. A low-powered laser then treats these vessels which are shown up by the dye. This means they are stopped from leaking and causing further damage. This treatment often needs to be repeated several times to prevent recurrence of the growth of these vessels. This type of treatment is known as PhotoDynamic Therapy (or PDT). While not a cure this therapy does prevent further loss of vision in some specific sufferers. People suitable for PDT need to be carefully selected as the treatment will only benefit people with a specific type of AMD – 'classic' AMD. The 'occult' form will not benefit.

Drug treatment has also been researched. Various drugs have been tried to stop the process of the formation of the abnormal blood vessels seen in AMD, but no specific drug has been found to be of any value. But again research into this aspect is continuing.

Surgery is also being researched and performed. In one form of surgery the healthy retina overlying the abnormal blood vessels is removed, and placed on another part of the eye which has no underlying abnormality. This is difficult, meticulous surgery and is as yet in its infancy. Again only a small number of people have the type of AMD which is suitable for this process.

The above is only a brief rundown of some of the work proceeding into the cause and treatment of this condition.

Other work continues into the advancement of low-vision aids, help with their use and promotion of the availability of such helpful pieces of equipment to sufferers from macular degeneration. The Macular Disease Society is at the forefront of these educational processes as well as prompting an evaluation of the impact of AMD on people and society in general.

Perhaps one day the full story of this disease will be unravelled and successful treatment will be available. Meanwhile, much can be done to assist with coping strategies for this unpleasant disease which does seem to be on the increase worldwide.

Summary

- Genetic research – some success with juvenile macular degeneration but not with AMD.
- Risk factors have been confirmed.
- Further laser treatment (PhotoDynamic Therapy), drugs and surgery are all being researched.
- Coping strategies continue to be investigated, evaluated and improved.

Glossary

Amsler Chart chart used to test for macular degeneration
Antioxidants substances capable of neutralizing free radicals
Aqueous humour watery fluid that fills the eye in front of the lens
Blind spot small area of retina where nerve fibres pass to the brain
Cataract opacity in lens of the eye
Cornea circular transparent part at the front of the eyeball
Diabetic retinopathy changes in the retina that can occur in diabetics
Drusen deposits found in retina in macular degeneration
Field of vision amount of vision found in the periphery
Floaters opacities in the vitreous humour
Glaucoma disease in which the pressure in the eyeball is raised
Insulin substance secreted by the pancreas which controls sugar metabolism
Iris coloured part of the eye that regulates the amount of light entering the eye
Lens transparent structure situated behind the pupil
Macula tiny yellow spot on retina that contains a greater concentration of cones
Macular hole condition when only a minute part of the retina is affected by macular degeneration
Ophthalmologist doctor specializing in eye conditions
Ophthalmoscope equipment used to examine the back of the eye
Optic nerve nerve responsible for conduction of impulses to the brain from the eye
Optometrist person testing vision and dispensing glasses (also known as an optician)

Orbit bony cavity in skull surrounding the eye

Pancreas organ in abdomen controlling sugar metabolism and assisting with digestion

Presbyopia difficulty in reading print at normal distance in older age group

Pupil central opening in the iris in front of the lens

Retina light-sensitive area at the back of the eye

Retinal detachment condition in which the retina separates from the underlying structures of the eye

Snellen Chart chart used to test distance vision – letters of differing sizes

Squint an abnormal alignment of the eyes

Stargardt's disease juvenile form of macular degeneration

Toxometry method of checking pressure in the eyeball

Vitreous humour transparent fluid that fills the eyeball behind the lens

Useful addresses

Disability Rights Commission (DRC)
DRC Helpline
FREEPOST MID02164
Stratford-upon-Avon
CV37 9BR
Tel.: 08457 622 633
Website: www.drc-gb.org

The Macular Disease Society
P.O. Box 1870
Andover
Hants SP10 9AD
Tel.: 01264 350551
Website: www.maculardisease.org

Partially Sighted Society
Queen's Road
Doncaster
S. Yorks DN1 2NX
Tel.: 01302 323132 or 01302 368998
Website: http://jim.leeder.users.btopenworld.com/LHON/
uk-pss.htm

Royal National Institute for the Blind (RNIB)
105 Judd Street
London WC1H 9NE
Tel.: 020 7388 1266
Website: www.rnib.org.uk

Talking Newspaper Association of the United Kingdom
National Recording Centre
Heathfield
E. Sussex TN21 0DB
Tel.: 01435 866102
Website: www.tnauk.org.uk

Index

Side View (journal) 52–3, 69
smoking 18, 86–8
social life 75–7
squints 4
Stargardt's disease 30, 35
sunlight 18–19, 24
support groups 34, 52–3
television:
  closed circuit 64
  magnification 63, 64
toxometry 44
vision:
  long-sightedness 16

short-sightedness 49
size, shapes and colours
  22–4
testing 30–2
visual loss:
  AMD as leading cause of
    13
  legal registration 77–8
  types of ix–x

Watts, Mark:
  *Cataract: What You Need
    to Know* 49